INTERPROFESSIONAL WORKING IN HEALTH AND SOCIAL CARE

Other titles

Pollard K.C., Thomas J. and Miers M. (2010) *Understanding Interprofessional Working in Health and Social Care: Theory and Practice.* Basingstoke: Palgrave Macmillan.

Sellman D. (2011) *What Makes a Good Nurse: Why the Virtues Are Important for Nurses.* London: Jessica Kingsley.

Sellman D. and Snelling P. (eds) (2010) *Becoming a Nurse: A Textbook for Professional Practice.* Harlow: Pearson Education.

Interprofessional Working in Health and Social Care

Professional Perspectives

Second Edition

Edited by

Judith Thomas, Katherine C. Pollard and Derek Sellman

palgrave
macmillan

First edition 2005
Reprinted ten times
Second edition published 2014 by
PALGRAVE MACMILLAN

Palgrave Macmillan in the UK is an imprint of Macmillan Publishers Limited,
registered in England, company number 785998, of Houndmills, Basingstoke,
Hampshire RG21 6XS.

Palgrave Macmillan in the US is a division of St Martin's Press LLC,
175 Fifth Avenue, New York, NY 10010.

Palgrave Macmillan is the global academic imprint of the above companies
and has companies and representatives throughout the world.

Palgrave® and Macmillan® are registered trademarks in the United States,
the United Kingdom, Europe and other countries

ISBN: 978–0–230–39343–1 paperback

This book is printed on paper suitable for recycling and made from fully
managed and sustained forest sources. Logging, pulping and manufacturing
processes are expected to conform to the environmental regulations of the
country of origin.

A catalogue record for this book is available from the British Library.

A catalog record for this book is available from the Library of Congress.

Printed and bound in Great Britain by
TJ International, Padstow

Contents

Acknowledgements and Dedication

We owe our gratitude to the students of the Faculty of Health and Applied Sciences, University of the West of England, Bristol from whom a request for a book of this nature was initially suggested. We are very grateful to all of the contributing authors who have enriched the book through the provision of distinctive perspectives on interprofessional working.

We would like to dedicate this edition of the book to Gillian Barrett who was the lead editor of the first edition. Gill was a highly valued colleague and we wish her a long and happy retirement.

Notes on Contributors

Jan Chianese MSc, TDCR, Senior Lecturer, Faculty of Health and Applied Sciences, UWE (University of the West of England, Bristol). Jan's interests are in oncology, radiotherapy practice, adult education and student support.

Susan Davis RN, RM, PGCAE, MSc in Public health (Health Promotion). Sue has a background in nursing and midwifery. She teaches at UWE on a range of modules relating to midwifery practice, teaching and assessing. She works as a midwife and supervises midwives. Her research interests lie in health promotion, collaborative working, breast feeding and supporting midwives in the workplace.

Anne-Laure Donskoy MPhil (Psych), MA, DESS, DERCAV, Survivor researcher in mental health, and research partner in health and social care at UWE. Her research interests include experiential accounts using qualitative methods. The subject of her MPhil focused on the first episode of self-wounding, using a narrative approach. Her activism focuses on human rights and ethics in mental health at local, national and European levels. She has authored peer-reviewed papers on user research and user participation in France and Belgium and has authored or co-authored chapters in the UK and in France.

Fiona M. Douglas MSc, DipCOT, DACE, Senior Lecturer and Occupational Therapy Programme Manager, Faculty of Health and Applied Sciences, UWE. Fiona's interests are in student centred learning, exploring and disseminating the concept of health and well-being through occupation, and multicultural concepts of education.

Lindsey Dow DM MSc (Medical Education), FRCP Consultant Geriatrician and Stroke Physician, Older People's Unit, Royal United Hospital Bath NHS Trust, Honorary Senior Clinical Lecturer, Bristol University. Lindsey's interests are medical education and health care in older people and stroke medicine. She lectures and delivers clinical ward based teaching to 6th formers, undergraduate medical students, junior doctors and general practitioners. She also teaches on the Bristol and Bath multiprofessional stroke education course.

Karen Dunmall MSc SRM (Open), BSc (Hons) (Open), Pg Cert HE, DCR(R), Programme Manager BSc(Hons) Diagnostic Imaging at UWE. Karen's interests are in teaching and learning styles of radiographers, radiography education, student and patient experience. Karen qualified as a diagnostic radiographer in 1980 and has worked in many departments throughout the UK and overseas.

Nansi Evans MBBCh, MRCGP, DCH, Dip Pall Med Work. Nansi works as a general practitioner, her interests include women's health, palliative medicine and medical humanities.

Robin Fletcher BA, MA, PhD is the Director of Programmes for the Department of Criminology and Sociology at Middlesex University. He is a retired Detective Superintendent whose PhD thesis examined Police Goverance and the introduction of the Crime and Disorder Act 1998. His pedagogic interests include British organised crime, the ethics and process of criminal investigations, and police education.

Matthew Godsell PhD, PGCE, RNT, RNLD, Senior Lecturer, Faculty of Health and Applied Sciences, UWE. Matthew's interests are the health of people with learning disabilities, nursing, social policy and historical perspectives on health and welfare.

Ken Holmes MSc DRI Cert CI. Programme Leader BSc(Hons) Diagnostic Radiography, University of Cumbria. Ken's interests are in the provision and assessment of clinical practice.

Karen Jones is a freelance trainer and consultant. She has worked extensively as a social work practitioner, educator and writer and has a particular interest in work with older people.

Celia Keeping MA, CQSW, Senior Lecturer, Faculty of Health and Applied Sciences, UWE. Until recently Celia worked in practice as a mental health social worker. She is particularly interested in relationship-based practice and is involved in skills development within social work education.

Peter Kennison BA, MA, PhD, is Senior Lecturer, Department of Criminology, University of Brighton. Peter's interests include police accountability, community safety and child protection. His PhD focused on policing diversity as seen through the police complaints system; he has also published on child protection and the Internet, police use of firearms, and understanding suicide terrorism in the light of the shooting of Jean Charles Menezes.

Jane Lindsay MA, MSc, CQSW, AASW, Acting Head of School, School of Social Work, Kingston University and St George's University of London and Probation Officer, London Probation Trust working on domestic abuse intervention programmes

Helen Martin MEd, BA (Hons), Cert. Ed., Dip. COT, Senior Lecturer at UWE. Helen's interests include interprofessional education, student learning on placements, and using creative activities with people with dementia.

Billie Oliver BEd (Hons), MEd, EdD, is Associate Professor for Integrated Children's and Young People's Services at UWE. A qualified Youth Worker, Billie's background includes working with children, young people and adults in community and voluntary sector settings. She has research interests in children's social policy, interprofessional working, professional identity and participatory community engagement.

Bob Pitt EdD, Senior Lecturer, Department of Health and Applied Social Sciences, UWE. Bob's professional background is in community and adult education and community work. He manages a programme for practitioners working with children, young people and their families. He teaches on social work and public health programmes at undergraduate and postgraduate level.

Katherine C. Pollard PhD, MSc, PGDip (SocSci), BA, Dip HEM (Midwifery), Senior Research Fellow, Faculty of Health and Applied Sciences, UWE. Her research interests include interprofessional education and practice, public and patient engagement and service evaluation in health and social care. She has authored numerous peer-reviewed articles about interprofessional learning and working, and her PhD, completed in 2007, focused on interprofessional working in maternity care.

Dianne Rees Bed (Hons), MA, EdD, MCSP, Associate Head of Department of Allied Health Professions, Faculty of Health and Applied Sciences, UWE. A physiotherapist by profession, Dianne has worked in higher education since 1992. Her research interests include academic staff views and experiences of interprofessional education in health and social care (HSC), and the application of Bourdieusian theory to HSC higher education. These formed the focus of her professional doctorate in education, which was completed in 2012.

Judith Ritchie BA (Hons), PGCE, MCIH, Senior Lecturer and Programme Leader, Faculty of the Built Environment, UWE. Judith's interests are in housing care and support and homelessness.

Kuljit Sandhu MA/Dipsw, BA (Hons), Assistant Chief Officer, London Probation Trust and Senior leader in development of a public sector mutual.

Kuljit's interests are preventive and rehabilitative interventions to reduce reoffending, effectiveness of what works and change management.

Derek Sellman PhD, RN, Associate Professor, Faculty of Nursing, University of Alberta. Derek's interests include education for professional practice, health care ethics, and philosophy of nursing.

Gary Smart BEd (Hons), MCPara, Programme Leader Paramedic Science, Senior Lecturer in Emergency and Critical Care, UWE. Gary's interests are in paramedic education and advanced trauma care.

Kevin Stone DipSW, GradDip, BSc (Hons), PGCert, is a Senior Lecturer in Social Work, Faculty of Health and Applied Sciences, UWE. His areas of interest include approved mental health practice and risk in social work practice. Prior to this he worked as an Approved Mental Health Practitioner, as a social worker in an Emergency Duty Team and as a locality Team Manager. He is currently undertaking a Doctoral degree in Social Science at the University of Bristol.

Jane Tarr PhD, Associate Head of Department for Education and Early Childhood, Department of Education, UWE. Jane is interested in the educational and social inclusion of more vulnerable children and young people and has published a book together with Diana Tsokova called Diverse Perspectives on Inclusive School Communities (Routledge 2012) which includes stories from a wide range of professionals working with children and young people.

Judith Thomas MEd, CQSW, Faculty of Health and Applied Sciences, UWE, Continuing Professional Development Manager for Social Work. Judith worked as a social worker before moving into professional education. She has researched and published in the areas of health, social care and legal education. She has a number of publications relating to interprofessional learning and working including e-learning resources commissioned by the Social Care Institute for Excellence.

Mervyn Townley MA, DipN, Dip NEd, RGN, RMN, RN (Child), Post Grad Dip CBT, Consultant Nurse, Specialist CAMHS, Aneurin Bevan Health Board and Honorary Fellow, University of South Wales. His special interests are the transition period from child to adult mental health and in particular the development of Youth Mental Health Services and the post registration education of CAMHS professionals.

Adrian Vatcher Senior Lecturer in Social Work, Faculty of Health and Applied Sciences, UWE. Adrian worked as a social worker in the statutory sector. His areas of interest include ethics and values, working with families, care management law and policy, and social work practice in international contexts.

Ceri Victory MSc, MA(Oxon), MCIH, Senior Lecturer and Programme Leader, Faculty of the Built Environment, UWE and Chair Designate at Elim

Housing Association. Her professional interests include supported housing, housing management and development and housing policy.

Julie Williams MSc, BA (Hons), PGCEA, ADM, RM, RN. Julie is a Senior Lecturer in Midwifery, Faculty of Health and Applied Sciences, UWE. Her research interests include the development of the individual into a midwife and her MSc thesis explored how and why individuals make the choice to become midwives. She has also worked with a colleague on a number of research projects and published around the use and availability of complementary therapies in the midwifery services.

Introduction

Judith Thomas, Katherine C. Pollard and Derek Sellman

The nature of health and social care is such that, for many, the quality of the service received is dependent upon how effectively different professionals work together. Developments in knowledge and innovation in approaches to service delivery have resulted in a high level of specialisation. This means that it is not possible for any one professional to have sufficient knowledge and skills to respond to the requirements of individuals, groups and communities in situations of complex need (Irvine, Kerridge, McPhee and Freeman 2002). This being so, professionals have a 'moral obligation' (Irvine *et al.* 2002: 208) to work interprofessionally in order to serve the best interests of the service user.

This book sets out to enable those engaged in the health and social care arena to develop an understanding of the nature and policy context of interprofessional working, to consider some of the complexities involved when professionals work collaboratively and to provide examples of interprofessional working in practice. Interprofessional working is important in a range of contexts and in this book we use the term 'health and social care' to include some professional groups (such as education and housing) that might not appear to fit into that category. Nevertheless, each considers interprofessional working where there are health or social care aspects. The book is therefore relevant to those thinking about their career, to students undertaking professional pre-qualifying programmes within health, social care, education, youth work, housing and criminal justice and to qualified professionals working within the areas of service delivery covered in the different chapters. Since the first edition of this book a companion publication, *Understanding Interprofessional Working in Health and Social Care: Theory and*

Practice (Pollard, Miers and Thomas 2010), has been published which explores in more depth, theories and issues relating to interprofessional working.

This second edition has been updated to reflect some of the developments and changes to policy and legislation. It also includes two new chapters: one on service user and carer perspectives and another on new and emerging roles. Following the structure of the first edition, the content is arranged in three main parts. Part I comprises three chapters and concerns the need for interprofessional working, the processes involved, and perspectives on interprofessional working from a service user. In Chapter 1, Pollard, Sellman and Thomas identify a range of factors that have prompted the move from a separate, uniprofessional focus on the delivery of professional services to a more integrated interprofessional approach. Historical developments in the structuring and organisation of health and social care services are considered, together with political and professional drivers for collaboration. The terminology around joint working is explored and evidence of effectiveness considered. In Chapter 2, Keeping explores some of the knowledge, attitudes and relational skills required to enable different professions to engage collaboratively. A number of difficulties that can arise within the context of interprofessional working are considered, together with a range of actions that can support those involved. Chapter 3 prompts us to think about service users and carers; it traces the development of law and policy that places them at the centre of services and any decisions made about their care and treatment and also questions the reality behind some of the rhetoric.

Part II contains 12 chapters, each one focusing on a particular profession. As knowledge regarding the existence and function of professions is a factor influencing interprofessional working, the authors of each chapter initially outline professional roles and responsibilities before citing examples of interprofessional working. Chapters are set out in the following alphabetical order: education, housing, medicine, midwifery, nursing, occupational therapy, physiotherapy, police, probation, radiography, social work and youth work. The overall aim of each of the 12 professions represented in the book is to provide benefit to individuals, groups or society in general. Yet the significant differences in their respective histories and trajectories results in profession-specific traditions in language use, to particular conventions regarding terminology and to differences in academic preparation. These differences provide a diversity of approach to health and social care practices reflected in the different ways in which chapter authors write about their profession and about its relationships both with other professions and with users of the service: so the reader will find a range of terms used by professionals to refer to the people for whom they provide services including, for example, service user, patient and client.

Case studies are used to illustrate interprofessional working in an intra-agency context (involving different professionals working within the same organisation/agency) and in a multiagency context (involving different professionals working across different organisational or agency boundaries). In the case studies fictitious names are used, except in Chapter 11 which focuses on Victoria Climbié and Peter Connelly. First names of people may be used for clarity and consistency. This is not meant to imply that in their interactions professionals and users of services will be on first name terms. In any relationship good professional practice involves ascertaining how people prefer to be addressed.

Chapter 3 identifies service users as experts in relation to their own needs and requirements, and Tarr's chapter on education (Chapter 4) illustrates the importance of involving carers within the collaborative process if a satisfactory outcome is to be achieved. Similarly the case study discussed by Vatcher and Jones (Chapter 14) highlights the need for professionals to work collaboratively with individual family members as well as with one another. Chapter 14 looks at social work and it is important to note the difference between social work, which is undertaken by qualified social workers in a clearly professionally regulated framework, and social care, which is a much broader term and covers a wider workforce.

There are occasions when, although collaborative working takes place between professionals, contact with the client is channelled through one professional adviser in order to ensure coherence across different agency boundaries. This is the nature of the interprofessional working discussed by Oliver and Pitt in their chapter on youth work (Chapter 15).

In Chapter 8 Sellman, Godsell and Townley cite the case of a mature male with moderate learning disabilities who suffers a heart attack, in order to illustrate the need for nurses to work collaboratively with other professionals in facilitating the smooth transition of service users between primary and secondary care. Collaboration between primary and secondary care professionals also forms the focus for the case study set out by Dow and Evans in their chapter on the role of doctors (Chapter 6). Dow and Evans consider multiprofessional, patient-held, records as a means of facilitating communication between the different professionals involved in the care of a man with acute and chronic health problems before discussing some of the difficulties that this might present.

The theme of smooth transition between different care settings is also evident in Williams and Davis's chapter on midwifery (Chapter 7). The authors outline the role of the midwife in supporting a pregnant woman with diabetes who is dependent on insulin, and discuss the need for collaborative working to ensure that her medical condition does not impact detrimentally on either her health and well-being or that of her baby.

Chapters 10 and 13 provide examples of interprofessional working within intra-agency contexts and detail the changing nature of the professional workforce resulting from the development of new career pathways. Rees's chapter on physiotherapy (Chapter 10) identifies the need for professionals to work collaboratively in order to provide a consistent approach to supporting the recovery of someone who has suffered a stroke. The context for Chapter 13 is a specialist oncology unit and Chianese, Dunmall and Holmes consider the contribution of the two radiography professions to the interprofessional team that supports a woman through the diagnosis and treatment of breast cancer.

Family relationships can sometimes be a source of emotional turmoil resulting in the need to support more than one family member at the same time. One of the case studies in Chapter 8 illustrates this and Sellman, Godsell and Townley identify the contribution of those involved in a child and adolescent mental health team in enabling different professionals to work with different family members in order to avoid a potential conflict of interest.

The probation service is the context for Chapter 12 in which Lindsay and Sandhu illustrate the contribution of interprofessional working to public safety. A case of domestic violence sets the scene to illustrate the contribution of probation and other services in developing an integrated approach to providing support to victims of abuse.

In Chapter 9 Douglas and Martin demonstrate the role of the occupational therapist in facilitating an interprofessional approach, which prevented a breakdown in service delivery to a young woman, Kim, with bipolar disorder who has a child. Here the occupational therapist needs to work with parents, social workers, mental health workers and community nurses as well as with Kim to support her in leading a more independent life and developing a safe and trusting relationship with her son.

The diversity of housing provision and the relationship between housing and health is highlighted in Chapter 5. Carlton and Ritchie use two case studies to illustrate some of the ways in which health care, social care and housing professionals can work in partnership for the benefit of individuals with housing needs.

Interprofessional working is fraught with difficulties and the cases of Victoria Climbié and baby Peter Connelly are used by Kennison and Fletcher in their chapter on the police (Chapter 11) to illustrate how lack of training, blurred roles, poor communication and poor quality supervision contribute to inadequate child protection. Sellman, Godsell and Townley in Chapter 8 highlight some of the complexities associated with operationalising interprofessional working at a time when a particular nursing service is in the process of transition.

Part III has two chapters. In Chapter 16, Thomas, Smart and Stone discuss new and emerging roles using the examples of the specialist paramedic and the approved mental health practitioner to consider some of the challenges of these roles and explore the uptake of these duties by people from different professional backgrounds. In the final chapter Thomas explores further some of the issues raised in earlier chapters. The case is made for critical reflection as a means to facilitate the development of the transferable team work skills required for effective interprofessional working.

The chapters include questions and activities designed to encourage the reader to reflect upon and think critically about identified aspects of interprofessional working. These questions are designed to enable readers to develop a personal action plan to foster the development of relevant knowledge, skills and attitudes to support their involvement in interprofessional working. The authors refer to relevant legislation giving the full title name of the Act and a reference to the website www.legislation.gov.uk so that readers can use the title and date of the Act to study it further and also identify whether the legislation applies to the whole of the United Kingdom or just to specific countries. Each of the chapters in Part II can only offer a glimpse into the role of the different professionals under discussion and we acknowledge that to give a true picture of each of the professions covered requires much more research and study. Thus authors have included recommendations for further reading to support and deepen readers' understandings of each of the professions and issues explored in each of the profession specific chapters.

The book also concentrates on interprofessional working rather than interprofessional education and although there are some references to interprofessional education the reader will need to explore other publications that cover the debates around the importance of learning about and with other professionals at all stages of their professional development. There are many helpful studies of interprofessional education, for example, Barr, Helme and D'Avray (2011), Le Riche and Taylor (2008) and Sharland and Taylor (2007), with other examples on the websites noted in the reference list below; in addition, the *Journal of Interprofessional Care* contains many other studies that are referenced within this book.

References

Barr H., Helme M. and D'Avray L. (2011) *Developing Interprofessional Education in Health and Social Care Courses in the United Kingdom*. Paper 12. The Higher Education Academy, Health Sciences and Practice. www.health.heacademy.ac.uk. Accessed June 2013.

Irvine R., Kerridge I., McPhee J. and Freeman S. (2002) Interprofessionalism and ethics: consensus or clash of cultures? *Journal of Interprofessional Care* 16: 199–210.

Le Riche P. and Taylor I. (2008) *The Learning, Teaching and Assessment of Partnership Work in Social Work Education SCIE Guide 23* www.scie.org.uk. Accessed July 2013.

Pollard K.C., Miers M. and Thomas J. (2010) *Understanding Interprofessional Working in Health and Social Care: Theory and Practice*. Basingstoke: Palgrave.

Sharland E. and Taylor I. (2007) *Interprofessional Education for Qualifying Social Work*. London: Social Care Institute for Excellence. www.scie.org.uk. Accessed July 2013.

PART I

Understanding Interprofessional Working

The Need for Interprofessional Working

Katherine C. Pollard, Derek Sellman and Judith Thomas

Introduction

This chapter traces developments in collaborative working and examines some of the reasons why interprofessional working is considered so crucial in the delivery of health and social care services. While recognising the increased emphasis that has been placed globally on the need for interprofessional working since the beginning of the 21st century, it should be recognised that collaboration and team working across professions has a considerably longer history.

The growth of the public sector in the United Kingdom (UK) since Victorian times is a history of the separate development of different professional and occupational groups. The birth and development of public sector professions and occupations may be interdependent in some ways but the rise in status of these occupational groups has not always benefited the public (Miller 2004). Service provision across the public sector was initially organised by separate professions and agencies. In the latter part of the 20th century an increasing awareness emerged regarding the need to link services and integrate methods of service delivery in order best to meet the stated objectives of public policy. From the late 1960s, policy documents reveal an increasing concern with the development of formal partnerships between different agencies as well as between professional groupings.

In this chapter, we will look at some of the factors that have given rise to the current prominence of interprofessional working. We will discuss common terminology and examine some of the related government policies and professional issues. As explained in the introduction there are some questions within the chapter to encourage you to develop your own ideas about interprofessional working. We also will consider some aspects of the position of patients/service users in relation to interprofessional working, although these are explored more fully in Chapter 3.

Health and social care in the United Kingdom

Before World War II, there was no national consistency in the standards or organisation of health and social care in the UK as services were provided by a mixture of charities, local civic bodies and independent professionals who charged for their services. The Labour government of the 1940s passed key legislation for education and for the provision of social care for children, older people, people with disabilities and homeless people, as well as establishing the National Health Service (NHS). Until the advent of Thatcherism in the 1980s the post-war consensus meant that health and social services were centrally financed, with differing degrees of local autonomy, while control of service delivery rested largely in the hands of the relevant professions (Allsop 1995, Gladstone 1995). This period was characterised by a relatively cohesive organisation of service delivery at a uniprofessional level, with varying and unpredictable degrees of interprofessional working. Each profession developed in its own way, with little shared tradition of interprofessional collaboration. Patients/service users were passive recipients of services, although acknowledgement that there should be channels through which they could have a voice was implicit in the establishment of the Community Health Councils in 1974 (Allsop 1995). Local government controlled social care services, so while the local democratic process had some impact on policy this rarely translated into changes in service delivery.

The economic, social and political changes of the Thatcher era in the 1980s resulted in a major reorganisation of all public services. The market emphasis on the consumer reinforced a developing civic awareness among the general public and led to demands for coherence, accountability and transparency from service providers. At the same time, the Conservative government of the day emphasised particularly tight controls over public expenditure. These conditions paved the way for the restructuring of public services in alignment with models for market-driven organisations, with an emphasis on cost-effectiveness and choice for the consumer. A major development of this era was the creation of the internal market, which resulted in some agencies and professions being assigned to a purchaser role, while others were designated as providers. So, for example, purchaser general practitioners (GPs) were permitted to buy acute services for their patients from provider NHS Trusts that ran the local hospital(s). Initiatives such as GP fundholding shifted financial control to local levels, with NHS Trusts operating as independent companies responsible for their own finances, free to sub-contract services and determine issues such as employment conditions for their staff independently. Similarly, some social services departments set up internal markets while others moved, willingly or not, into purchasing some of their care provision from other agencies (Allsop 1995, Gladstone 1995).

One important consequence of these changes was the shift of control of service delivery away from health and social care professionals (who had not previously been required to take account of the wider financial implications of service provision) to management bodies and managers. Management's main responsibility became to provide cost-effective services in line with government policy objectives. Another consequence of these changes was the increased fragmentation in the organisation of service delivery (Allsop 1995, Payne 2000). The negative consequences which can result from a system which has neither cohesive structures for service delivery nor effective interprofessional collaboration have been well documented; see, for example, Dalley (1993) and the Audit Commission (2000). Increasingly, the solution to these problems focused on the need for integration of services, an essential feature of which is collaborative working. Interprofessional working was also thought to be cost-effective in streamlining delivery systems and avoiding duplication (Paul and Peterson 2001) although a counter argument suggested that financial constraints can militate against the implementation and maintenance of interprofessional collaboration (Freeth 2001). A systematic review by Cameron, Lart, Bostock and Coomber sought to find evidence of the cost-effectiveness of interprofessional working but identified that 'Assessing the costs and cost-effectiveness of joint working is hampered by a lack of economic evaluation evidence, evidence that is dated and the diversity of approaches to integrating services' (2012: 7); so the answer to the question as to whether interprofessional working saves money is unclear.

The introduction of the private sector to provide services that were historically the responsibility of the public or statutory sector further transformed the public services landscape. For example, the private finance initiative (PFI), introduced in the early 1990s, has now become embedded in communities across the UK. Through PFI, a system was implemented whereby the private sector became jointly responsible with the public sector for the management and delivery of services in health care, education and the prison system, as well as owning buildings and equipment central to service delivery (Allen 2001). As time has passed, it is clear that, not only has this initiative moved control even further away from the hands of professionals, it has also contributed significantly to the financial difficulties in which many public sector organisations currently find themselves (Clark 2012). However, Cardy (2010) suggests that the increasing privatisation of health and social care in the UK appears inevitable. The 2012 Health and Social Care Act (www.legislation.gov.uk) paved the way for private companies to be more involved in providing services, as predicted by Peedell (2011). However, social enterprises or services that reinvest profits in the business in order to benefit the community are also becoming increasingly important providers of health and social care services (SCIE 2012).

Running in parallel with these managerial and economic changes has been the growing recognition that patients/service users have rights to information and to involvement in the planning and prioritisation of services. In 1991, the government established the Citizen's Charter Unit to document and disseminate the rights of consumers (that is, the public) as they relate to various fields of public sector activity, and 33 Citizens' Charters had been published by

1993. One of these was the Patient's Charter (DH 1992), which set standards for providers to meet for certain aspects of health care delivery. This charter ostensibly gives the public control and choice about the care they receive, although the extent to which these principles are actually applied in practice remains questionable twenty years after its publication (Simmons, Birchall and Prout 2012). However, whatever the gaps between rhetoric and reality, the legacy of the changes in health and social care in the UK over the last three decades is an emphasis on cost-effective integrated services that meet the needs of, and actively involve, patients/service users (see, for example, Bellis, Hughes, Perkins and Bennett 2012).

QUESTIONS

- What developments were you already aware of in the section above?
- What information was new to you?
- What do you think interprofessional working involves?
- How do you think the way in which services are developing impact on your understanding of interprofessional working?

The next section will help you think more about the meaning of the term interprofessional working and as you read through other chapters in the book refer back to your answers to the questions above and add any other thoughts that are relevant to the questions.

What is interprofessional working?

Interprofessional working requires that personnel from different professions and agencies work together. There has been extended debate about terminology in this field. Readers will find, among others, the terms multiprofessional, interprofessional, multidisciplinary, interdisciplinary, multiagency and interagency being used to describe what appear to be very similar activities. A broad rule of thumb is that the prefix *multi* tends to indicate the involvement of personnel from different professions, disciplines or agencies, but does not necessarily imply collaboration. The prefix *inter* tends to imply collaboration, particularly in areas such as decision-making (Øvretveit 1997, Payne 2000). One way of conceptualising interprofessional work is in terms of the effectiveness of coordination and communication. Social workers, for example, have traditionally emphasised the importance of coordination of services where more than one agency or worker is involved. This occurs in areas such as key aspects of mental health work, community care, and in child protection.

Team is another term which is often used when describing working groups; however, what is meant (and understood) by this word can vary enormously. Teams may be tightly knit units, composed of individuals who regularly work together; or they may be loosely woven entities which emerge in an *ad hoc* manner to meet specific demands. A team may just be a convenient way of describing a group of staff with a common manager but with little else that brings them together. Teams may be formally constituted, with a specified structure and objective, or they may arise organically with no formal recognition. They may be consensual, democratic or hierarchical in nature, or all of these by turn, depending on circumstances. The members of a team may collaborate with one another in practice, or they may act alone on behalf of the team. Teams may draw their members from a single professional group, or from several. These are only some of the variations that can be found, in many different permutations, in team structure and process (Øvretveit 1997, Payne 2000).

ACTIVITY

Before you read the next paragraph make a note of what you understand by collaborative working and compare your thoughts with the ideas below.

In this book, we take interprofessional working to mean collaborative practice: that is, the process whereby members of different professions and/or agencies work with each other and with patients/service users, to provide integrated health and/or social care for the latter's benefit. This definition is consistent with that of Wood and Gray: 'Collaboration occurs when a group of autonomous stakeholders of a problem domain engage in an interactive process, using shared rules, norms, and structures, to act or decide on issues relating to that domain' (1991: 146). The structure and logistics of the systems through which professionals organise their collaborative efforts vary considerably, in part influenced by the history of each profession or service, but are often crucially dictated by government policy and directive. Collaborative practice might take place through a single team of mixed professionals or through different organisations cooperating in planning and providing services. Since 2000, various governmental strategies have resulted in the development of new organisational forms thought to advance collaborative practice. An increasing emphasis on patient and public involvement (PPI) in the planning and delivery of health and social care services has resulted in a growing awareness of the need to involve patients/service users actively in processes regarding their own care (see Chapter 3).

Political drivers for interprofessional working

Reference to interprofessional working can be found in the USA in the medical and nursing literature of the 1960s, so the idea of collaborative practice is not new. For example:

> One hospital is reported to have weekly interprofessional ward conferences attended by all members of the clinical team.
>
> (Henderson 1966: 8)

In the UK, reference to interprofessional issues began to appear in the health and social care literature approximately a decade later; see, for example, Black (1977) and Dingwall (1977). The emergence of these ideas did not mean, however, that collaborative practice was necessarily a reality at this time.

Since the late 1970s, health and social care policy in most European countries has been based on meeting the World Health Organisation targets for improving health, contained in the Health for All Declaration of Alma-Ata (WHO 1978). During this period the European Union placed an emphasis on a right of parity for the health and social care of all citizens of member states, thus locating responsibility for the organisation of care with policy makers, answerable to the general public through the democratic process (Thompson and Mathias 1997). In the UK, this highlighted the tensions between professional autonomy in service delivery on the one hand and the edicts of central governmental control of professional working on the other, illustrated by the introduction of key directives including, for example, the Department of Health's (DH's) requirement that health and social care professionals provide evidence-based practice.

A chronological examination of UK policies between the late 1990s and the early years of the 21st century reveals explicit support for the premise that collaborative practice will improve the quality of service delivery. Continued emphasised on this feature can be found in the recent mandate issued by the government to the NHS Commissioning Board (DH 2012).

Some policy documents targeted specific professions. Making a Difference (DH 1999) stated explicitly that nurses, midwives and health visitors were expected to engage in interprofessional practices. This stance was reinforced in a document published in 2000, in which arrangements for workforce planning were criticised for not being:

> Holistic in their approach, looking across primary, secondary and tertiary care or across staff groups.
>
> (DH 2000: 19)

As time elapsed, many policy documents outline planned services whose success appeared to be entirely dependent upon effective interprofessional working. For example, the Department of Health, which also sets out the need for more personalised services that will be discussed later in this chapter, stated that:

> People with long-term conditions will be supported to manage their conditions themselves with the right help from health and social care services... To support a more integrated approach we will develop Personal Health and Social Care Plans and integrated social and health care records. To help people receive a more joined-up service, we will be establishing joint health and social care teams to support people with ongoing conditions who have the most complex needs.
>
> (DH 2006: 8)

It is obvious that these targets could only be met if health and social care workers were working well together. However, the situation on the ground was far from clear-cut, with accounts of both effective and difficult interprofessional working still being reported (see, for example, Pullon 2008). This situation was recognised in a key report led by Lord Darzi (DH 2008) which once again emphasised the need for good interprofessional working in health and social care. This emphasis was also found in a report published by the General Social Care Council in the same year, which stressed that developing partnerships is a core component of the social work role (GSCC 2008). In its turn, a policy document published two years later highlighted the importance of partnership working, particularly between public health and social services, for effective care delivery (DH 2010) and the 2012 Professional Capabilities Framework for social workers expects them to 'Operate effectively within multi-agency and inter-professional settings' (CSW 2012: 2). The Department of Health continues to send a similar message, particularly in recognition of the increase of long-term conditions:

> Too many people with ongoing health problems are treated as a collection of symptoms not a person. ... We need the NHS to do much better for people with long-term conditions or disabilities in the future ... different parts of the NHS have to work more effectively with each other and with other organisations, such as social services, to drive joined-up care.
>
> (DH 2012: 9)

The growth of managerialism is also inextricably linked to the interprofessional agenda. Thatcherism promoted the cult of the manager in part as a way of bringing private sector practices into the public sector; this perspective was maintained during the period during which New Labour was in power, and continues to hold sway under the current Conservative-Liberal Democrat coalition. Managerialism is thought to hold the promise of tackling waste and improving performance, and to be a way of tackling the inefficiencies of professional workers and trade unions. It is interesting to note that this stance has been adopted by governments of all persuasions over the last three decades.

Professional drivers for interprofessional working

A central aspect of interprofessional working concerns the relative power of different professional groups. Until fairly late in the 20th century, some (predominantly male) occupational groups were identified as professions. Professions were thought to include those pursuing a particular occupation by completion of a recognised course of education, typically at least to graduate level. Furthermore, they operated autonomously in their sphere of practice, were self-regulating and free from bureaucratic or managerial control (Witz 1992). By contrast, other (predominantly female) occupational groups were considered to be semi-professions, with training rather than education, regulation by members of other occupational groups and with working practices overseen by other professionals or by managers and bureaucrats. In the health and social care arena, only medical practitioners were seen to belong to a profession; members of other occupational groups, for example, allied health professionals, nurses, social workers and midwives, were all considered to belong to semi-professions. The medical profession was accordingly the dominant professional group in health and social care for most of the 20th century (Witz 1992).

It has been argued that among the principles of effective interprofessional collaboration are power sharing and parity, which enable people to have a real say in decisions which affect their work (Meads and Ashcroft 2005). Some authors have suggested the drive toward collaborative practice has provided members of the semi-professions with an opportunity to raise the status of their own occupational group, and to increase their share of occupational power (Kesby 2002). If interprofessional working is seen as a method of redistributing power, it seems the medical profession has most to lose. Interprofessional relationships are often complex, and allow investigation from a variety of perspectives: for example, the feminist tradition insists that gender relations are key to understanding interaction between professions and semi-professions (Witz 1992). Some of the problems of implementing interprofessional working among professionals whose priorities for advancing their own profession are not necessarily complementary will be discussed in Chapter 2.

The effect of interprofessional working on service delivery

There is a general consensus among health and social care professionals that integrated care, with its emphasis on effective collaborative practice, can improve services for users. There is evidence that a failure of collaboration can have tragic consequences (Kennedy 2001, Laming 2003, 2009) and the breakdown in communication between professionals is a common theme of child protection inquiries. The lack of collaborative practice between agencies and professionals is seen as being responsible for individual tragedies as well as for the failure to tackle general social problems such as social exclusion, homelessness, and crime and disorder (see, for example, Chapter 11). The principles of personalisation emphasise a need for all public services including transport, housing and leisure to work together to tackle these sorts of problems (SCIE 2012).

Despite the widespread assumption that successful interprofessional working will prevent such tragedies and poor practice, the evidence base remains sparse. There is little research directly investigating the effectiveness of collaborative practice in terms of outcomes for patients/service users. A few studies conducted in the 1990s did show that effective interprofessional working improved the quality of care provided (see, for example, Dawson and Bartlett 1996). It is worth noting that this and other relevant studies from that period were conducted in dedicated health care settings, for example, a closed psychiatric facility, where closely knit teams of professionals routinely worked alongside each other. The process of evaluating the outcomes of collaborative practice is more difficult in areas of service provision that require coordination between personnel from different organisations and agencies who interact infrequently. The concept of interprofessional working is imprecise, and different interpretations have led many researchers to concentrate on issues more easily accessible to evaluation.

The lack of research in this area, in contrast to the plethora of general literature concerning interprofessional issues, underlines how difficult it is to provide evidence to support the idea that collaborative practice improves service delivery. The nature of research requires that all variables affecting a process under investigation be considered. There are many variables in the delivery of public services and the way in which they interact is complex. Relevant contributing factors include: the amount and quality of social support, the composition of the interprofessional group, the way in which members of the group work together, the physical environment and the nature of interventions. For this reason isolation of effective interprofessional working as a definitive factor affecting the outcomes of service delivery is challenging at best. However, there is some logic in concluding that collaborative practice does generally improve the provision of services. The evidence base to support this claim is increasing (Cameron *et al.* 2012 and Dickinson 2008) and studies by Siassakos, Fox, Hunt *et al.* (2011) and Pollard, Miers and Rickaby (2012) suggest that not only are patients/service users and professionals often more satisfied where there is effective and relevant interprofessional collaboration but also that professionals consider that it substantively improves the quality of care.

Whether interprofessional working is always required remains a matter of debate. Despite the current rhetoric, it would be naive to consider interprofessional working as a panacea. It is possible that collaborative practice might encourage an abdication of personal responsibility. There are occasions when a specific professional perspective is appropriate for providing optimum service delivery. Where interprofessional processes and considerations are prioritised these occasions may pass unrecognised, with the potential for detrimental effects on individual patients/service users. Over time, this could result in a dilution of professional knowledge and skills. However, these potential negatives might result from poor interprofessional practice rather than be an unforeseen consequence of good practice. The judicious use and development of protocols that establish clear boundaries for decision making can aid in maintaining and increasing the skills repertoire of staff (Miers 2010). Overall we conclude that collaborative practice appears to hold out the promise of a positive impact on service delivery; however, the manner of implementation remains a crucial issue.

Service user involvement in interprofessional working

The current social and political climate demands that patients/service users are involved in the planning and prioritisation of service delivery (DH 2005, 2010, 2012). Government rhetoric promotes the principles of choice and control for users within a seamless service. Increasingly, the concept of interprofessional working is understood to include all stakeholders, whether patients/service users, carers, members of the public or professionals, particularly in the fields of mental health and social care. The Social Care Institute for Excellence (www.scie.org.uk) explicitly draws service users into the social care knowledge base and the service user perspective is being emphasised in all courses leading to qualification for health and social care practice. As early as 1998, it was proposed that:

> Health Action Zones will bring together a partnership of health organisations, including primary care, with Local Authorities, community groups, the voluntary sector and local businesses.
>
> (DH 1998: 43)

Although it took some time, the structures through which partnerships are to be established have become clearer over the intervening years (Bellis *et al.* 2010, Beresford 2010). While authentic (as opposed to 'token') service user involvement in decision making may still have not been achieved in some services, there has been noticeable progress in the development of suitable partnerships.

In terms of individual support since the 1990s, successive governments have promoted a policy agenda that has placed a growing emphasis on choice, independence and service user control, exercised within a more 'personalised' system of social work and social care. Direct Payments to enable people in need of social care services to purchase and manage their own care were introduced in 1997 and extended a few years later. This was seen as a significant victory for disability rights campaigners and reflected a wider policy trend towards choice and consumer rights.

Government papers (DH 2006, 2007, 2012) heralded another major shift towards more personalised services. The move towards 'self-directed support' which began with Direct Payments is central to the personalisation agenda. Self-directed support now commonly takes the form of a 'personal budget' – an amount of money allocated to meet the assessed needs of a person who is eligible for social care support. The money can be paid directly to the service user or to a trusted third party as a direct payment; alternatively it can be administered by the local authority or by a combination of the two.

Personalisation can be seen as an opportunity to work in more creative and empowering ways with service users and to offer effective, individualised assessments to meet the needs of carers. At the same time, however, there are concerns that financial constraints and tight eligibility criteria are increasingly restricting the range of services available to adults in need of support. The Social Care Institute for Excellence suggests that, among other things, personalisation means 'finding new collaborative ways of working (sometimes known as "co-production") that support people to actively engage in the design, delivery and evaluation of services' (SCIE 2012: 2).

Conclusion

Changes in the UK health and welfare context in the final two decades of the 20th century, most notably the establishment of the internal market, coupled with traditional professional 'territorial' attitudes, resulted in the fragmentation of the delivery of health and social care services, with detrimental effects for some service users. A perceived solution to this problem, particularly since the start of the 21st century, has been the development of integrated services, which require members of different professions and agencies to work together for the benefit of patients/service users. This emphasis on collaborative practice has been further driven by the need for services to be cost-effective on the assumption that, by preventing duplication of provision, integrated care requires fewer resources.

Successive governments have positioned collaborative practice as a cornerstone of effective integrated service delivery. Professional responses to this development have varied, influenced by issues of power and differing professional agendas. Increasingly, it is assumed that collaborative practice must involve not only professionals but also patients/service users, so that the latter are actively involved in the planning and prioritisation of services.

<hr>

RECOMMENDED READING

▦ Department of Health (2008) *High Quality Care for All: NHS next stage review final report.* Chair, Lord Darzi. CM 7432. London: The Stationery Office.

▦ Dickinson H. (2008) *Evaluating Outcomes in Health and Social Care.* Bristol: Policy Press.

▦ Meads G. and Ashcroft J., with Barr H., Scott R. and Wild A. (2005) *The Case for Interprofessional Collaboration in Health and Social Care.* Oxford: Blackwell.

<hr>

References

Allen G. (2001) *The Private Finance Initiative (PFI): Research Paper 01/117.* London: House of Commons Library.

Allsop J. (1995) Health: From seamless service to patchwork quilt. In Gladstone D. (ed.) *British Social Welfare: Past, Present and Future.* London: UCL Press, pp. 98–123.

Audit Commission (2000) *The Way to Go Home: Rehabilitation and Remedial Services for Older People.* London: The Stationery Office.

Bellis M.A., Hughes K., Perkins C. and Bennett A. (2012) *Protecting People, Promoting Health: A Public Health Approach to Violence Prevention for England.* www.preventviolence.info (accessed November 2012).

Beresford P. (2010) Public partnerships, governance and user involvement: A service user perspective. *International Journal of Consumer Studies* **34**(5): 495-502.

Black P (1977) The child at risk-interprofessional co-operation. *Nursing Mirror and Midwives Journal* **144**(15): 61–4.

Cameron A., Lart R., Bostock L. and Coomber C. (2012) *Research Briefing 41: Factors that Promote and Hinder Joint and Integrated Working between Health and Social Care Services.* London: SCIE.

Cardy S. (2010) 'Care Matters' and the privatization of looked after children's services in England and Wales: Developing a critique of independent 'social work practices'. *Critical Social Policy* **30**(3): 430–42.

Clark R. (2012) Paying for PFI: Labour's financial fudge is killing the NHS. *Spectator* **319**(9592): 18.

CSW (College of Social Work) (2012) *Domains within the PCF.* www.collegeofsocialwork.org/ (accessed February 2013).

Dalley G. (1993) Professional ideology or organisational tribalism? The health service-social work divide. In Walmsley J., Reynolds J., Shakespeare P. and Woolfe R. (eds) *Health, Welfare and Practice: Reflections on Roles and Relationships.* Buckingham: Open University Press, pp. 32–9.

Dawson J. and Bartlett E. (1996) Change within interdisciplinary teamwork: One unit's experience. *British Journal of Therapy and Rehabilitation* **3**: 219–22.

DH (Department of Health) (1992) *The Patient's Charter.* London: DH.

DH (1998) *Our Healthier Nation – A Contract for Health: A Consultation Paper.* London: The Stationery Office.

DH (1999) *Making a Difference: Strengthening the Nursing, Midwifery and Health Visiting Contribution to Health and Healthcare.* London: DH.

DH (2000) *A Health Service of All the Talents: Developing the NHS Workforce. Consultation Document on the Review of Workforce Planning.* London: DH.

DH (2005) *Creating a Patient Led NHS – Delivering the NHS Improvement Plan.* London: The Stationery Office.

DH (2006) *Our Health, Our Care, Our Say: A New Direction for Community Services.* London: DH.

DH (2007) *Putting People First: A Shared Vision and Commitment to the Transformation of Adult Social Care.* London: The Stationery Office.

DH (2008) *High Quality Care for All: NHS Next Stage Review Final Report.* Chair, Lord Darzi. CM 7432. London: The Stationery Office.

DH (2010) *Equity and Excellence: Liberating the NHS.* Norwich: The Stationery Office.

DH (2012) *The Mandate: A Mandate from the Government to the NHS Commissioning Board: April 2013 to March 2015.* London: DH.

Dickinson H. (2008) *Evaluating Outcomes in Health and Social Care.* Bristol: Policy Press.

Dingwall R. (1977) *The Social Organisation of Health Visiting Training.* London: Croom Helm.

Freeth D. (2001) Sustaining interprofessional collaboration. *Journal of Interprofessional Care* **15**: 37–46.

GSCC (General Social Care Council) (2008) *Social Work at its Best: A Statement of Social Work Roles and Tasks for the 21ˢᵗ Century.* www.gscc.org.uk/ (accessed November 2012).

Gladstone D. (1995) Individual welfare: Locating care in the mixed economy. Introducing the personal social services. In Gladstone D. (ed.) *British Social Welfare: Past, Present and Future.* London: UCL Press, pp. 161–70.

Henderson V. (1966) *The Nature of Nursing: A Definition and its Implications for Practice, Research, and Education.* New York: Macmillan.

Kennedy I. (2001) *Learning from Bristol: The Report of the Public Inquiry into Children's Heart Surgery at the Bristol Royal Infirmary 1984–1995.* London: The Stationary Office.

Kesby S. (2002) Nursing care and collaborative practice. *Journal of Clinical Nursing* **11**: 357–66.

Laming, Lord (2003) Inquiry into the Death of Victoria Climbié. London: The Stationary Office.

Laming, Lord (2009) *The Protection of Children in England: A Progress Report.* Norwich: The Stationery Office.

Meads G. and Ashcroft J. (2005) Policy into practice: Collaboration. In Meads G. and Ashcroft J., with Barr H., Scott R. and Wild A., *The Case for Interprofessional Collaboration in Health and Social Care.* Oxford: Blackwell, pp. 15–35.

Miers M. (2010) Learning for new ways of working. In Pollard K.C., Thomas J. and Miers M. (eds) *Understanding Interprofessional Working in Health and Social Care: Theory and Practice.* Basingstoke: Palgrave, pp. 74–89.

Miller C. (2004) *Producing Welfare: A Modern Agenda.* Basingstoke: Palgrave.

Øvretveit J. (1997) How to describe interprofessional working. In Øvretveit J., Mathias P. and Thompson T. (eds) *Interprofessional Working for Health and Social Care.* Basingstoke: Macmillan, pp. 9–33.

Paul S. and Peterson Q. (2001) Interprofessional collaboration: Issues for practice and research. *Occupational Therapy in Health Care* **15**(3/4): 1–12.

Payne M. (2000) *Teamwork in Multiprofessional Care.* Basingstoke: Macmillan.

Peedell C. (2011) Further privatisation is inevitable under the proposed NHS reforms. *British Medical Journal* **342**: 2996.

Pollard K., Miers M. and Rickaby C. (2012) 'Oh why didn't I take more notice?' Professionals' views and perceptions of their pre-qualifying interprofessional learning as preparation for inter-professional working in practice. *Journal of Interprofessional Care* **26**(5): 355–61.

Pullon S. (2008) Competence, respect and trust: Key features of successful interprofessional nurse-doctor relationships. *Journal of Interprofessional Care* **22**(2): 133–47.

SCIE (Social Care Institute for Excellence) (2012) *Personalisation: A rough guide: Guide 47.* London: SCIE.

Siassakos D., Fox R., Hunt L., Farey J., Laxton C., Winter C. and Draycott T. (2011) Attitudes toward safety and teamwork in a maternity unit with embedded team training. *American Journal of Medical Quality* **26**(2): 132–7.

Simmons R., Birchall J. and Prout A. (2012) User involvement in public services: 'Choice about voice'. *Public Policy and Administration* **27**(1): 3–29.

Thompson T. and Mathias P. (1997) The World Health Organisation and European Union: Occupational, vocational and health initiatives and their implications for cooperation amongst the professions. In Øvretveit J., Mathias P. and Thompson T. (eds) *Interprofessional Working for Health and Social Care*. Basingstoke: Palgrave, pp. 201–25.

WHO (World Health Organisation) (1978) *Primary Health Care: Report of the International Conference on Primary Health Care, Alma-Ata, USSR, 6–12 September 1978. (Health for All Series No. 1)*. Geneva: WHO.

Witz A. (1992) *Professions and Patriarchy*. London: Routledge.

Wood D.J. and Gray B. (1991) Towards a comprehensive theory of collaboration. *Journal of Applied Behavioural Science* **27**: 139–62.

The Processes Required for Effective Interprofessional Working

Celia Keeping

Introduction

Interprofessional working involves complex interactions between two or more members of different professional disciplines. It is a collaborative venture (McCray 2002) in which those involved share the common purpose of developing mutually negotiated goals achieved through agreed plans that are monitored and evaluated. The context within which this process is undertaken is important to consider as various dominant political and social discourses will significantly affect the identification, attainment and evaluation of these goals. Therefore, although this chapter concentrates on individual practitioners and their immediate colleagues, the actions, thoughts and feelings of these actors are understood as being influenced by the political, social and organisational context in which they operate.

Although the current health and social care policy agenda is advocating interprofessional and interagency working, policy directives alone are insufficient to ensure the desired outcome (Cameron 2011). As individuals, each member of the partnership needs to actively engage with the business of collaboration. They will need to be members of a supportive organisation which actively and effectively coordinates and manages relationships with other organisations and professional groups on a higher level. The failure of agencies to work together at a senior manager level will have major implications for how individual practitioners work together in the field.

Bearing this in mind, however, this chapter explores some of the processes which are likely to enable and encourage individual professionals to work together collaboratively. It will suggest that each member of the interprofessional endeavour needs to possess a set of particular skills and abilities if person-centred collaborative practice is to be a success. According to Suter, Arndt, Arthur *et al.* (2009) 'active ingredients' of collaboration fall into three conceptual domains: 'knowledge', 'attitudes' and 'relational skills'. These three domains are likewise referred to in the Interprofessional Capability Framework (Sheffield Hallam University 2010) as constituting key elements within four identified areas of learning designed to support and develop the individual in their capacity to work collaboratively. These four areas are collaborative working, reflection, cultural awareness and ethical practice, and organisational competence.

The chapter also considers some of the barriers to effective partnership working and, lastly, some suggestions are offered to support effective interprofessional working on an organisational level.

It should be noted that working effectively in an interprofessional context is a highly complex process. This chapter serves only as an introduction to this process, and wider reading is recommended for deeper appreciation of relevant issues and strategies.

Knowledge

Knowledge of professional roles

In order to provide a comprehensive approach to care a thorough holistic assessment of client needs is required. This necessitates a vision extending beyond the remit of a single profession or agency (Hornby and Atkins 2000, Pollard, Thomas and Miers 2010) and a perception that encompasses the scope of all professionals who might contribute to meeting the needs of particular service users. Ignorance of the existence and function of other professions and agencies limits both communication and relationships within the interprofessional team and with the client themselves (Hall 2005, Irvine, Kerridge and Freeman 2002). Therefore, even when a comprehensive assessment is undertaken, unless individual practitioners are well informed regarding the role, performance (Willumsen, Ahgren and Odegard 2012) and professional boundaries of other professions, they may fail to engage with those who could make a valuable contribution to the interprofessional team. This knowledge should be complemented by an understanding of the legal frameworks, statutory and regulatory requirements of the professions that make up the practice team (Willumsen *et al.* 2012). The Interprofessional Capability Framework (Sheffield Hallam University 2010) endorses the view that profession-specific knowledge and underpinning ethical values should be shared across communities of practice in order to enhance collaborative working processes.

Learning

Many of the following chapters refer to case studies where individuals have complex needs which can only be met by a range of different professional interventions. For instance, Chapter 6 tells the story of Gregory Fitzpatrick, an 84-year-old man whose needs led to involvement not just by his GP and local hospital, but also by a social worker, occupational therapist, physiotherapist and practice nurse. Chapter 8 likewise uses a case study of a 15-year-old girl, Theresa, who has been admitted to hospital following an overdose of paracetamol tablets. Her needs cannot be met by ward staff alone and require the help of a specialist nurse from the Children and Adolescent Mental Health Services, a psychiatrist and a social worker. In order to help clarify understanding of the range of potential partners in the interprofessional project, the following chapters will outline basic details relating to the roles and task of different professional groups.

An expectation that individual practitioners be well-informed regarding professional roles and boundaries presupposes that these aspects of professional work are clearly defined, whereas in reality, this may not always be the case. Chapter 11 for example, refers to the Laming Report (2003) which found that confusion surrounding the roles, responsibilities and boundaries of police and social services led to ineffective interprofessional working practices with tragic consequences for 8-year-old Victoria Climbié. Similar concerns were noted in the more recent enquiry into the death of Peter Connelly (Local Safeguarding Children Board 2009). Brown, Lewis, Ellis *et al.* (2011) found that role boundary issues were blurred in a Primary Health Care Trust and the team lacked understanding of the scope of practice of other professionals. Both factors caused unhelpful conflict within the interdisciplinary team and the study found that resolution of this conflict was inhibited by lack of time and high workload, inequities in power, lack of motivation and fear of causing emotional distress. While some conflict, if worked through and resolved, can prove beneficial to team functioning, unresolved conflict can inhibit the interprofessional task and impact on the quality of service provided. Advances in professional practice and new developments in health and social care provision, mean that traditional roles are being transformed and new or extended roles are being developed, many of which involve cross-professional and cross-agency working (Cameron 2011). It may take some time for those involved in such developments to define their new roles and delineate their boundaries; uncertainty regarding the perimeters of professional roles can be a factor in limiting the utilisation of relevant professionals within interprofessional initiatives as discussed in Chapter 16. In order to operate within this uncertain environment it is often necessary to work flexibly, and negotiate new roles and boundaries.

Knowledge of policy developments

Public services in Great Britain and beyond are undergoing fundamental changes in their structure, mode of operation and remit with inevitable consequences for the nature of the professional task, not least the move towards interprofessional collaboration (Nancarrow and Borthwick 2005). An understanding of the political and economic context and resulting policy development is essential if professionals are to understand the changes being required of them. Boundary disputes common in interprofessional working (Cameron 2011) could be mitigated and the interprofessional project facilitated if greater clarity of the drivers was achieved and demands for change contextualised.

Attitudes

Willing participation

According to Pecukonis, Doyle and Bliss (2008) the first and most important step in the development of interprofessional collaboration is a willingness to engage with other professional groups. This willingness is likely to be linked to a viewpoint that values the ideologies of user-centred services and holistic care (Freeth 2001) as discussed in Chapter 3. Where this moral obligation to focus on the client is present, concerns relating to membership of a particular professional group are more likely to be transcended in the interests of collaborative working and the pursuit of the common goal of client care. This driving altruistic force 'is based on a concern for others and for the society at large' (Axelsson and Axelsson 2009: 324). For Sellman (2010) the willingness to collaborate includes a number of factors: acknowledgement of the contributions of other professionals (a sentiment shared by Axelsson and Axelsson 2009), a willingness to acknowledge personal limitations and an openness to engage in dialogue with different points of view. Above all, he considers that professionals must be willing to maintain and develop their skills in order to be able to maximise their contribution to the interprofessional endeavour.

In order to foster a sense of altruism and willingness to collaborate certain conditions need to be present relating to structure, culture and procedure. Kvarnstrom (2008) pointed out the problems caused by an unsupportive organisation and Keeping and Barrett (2009) suggest that if the organisation fails to provide a robust and thoughtful environment where principles of respect and safety exist, practitioners are unlikely to move away from old patterns of 'silo' thinking.

Trust and mutual respect

Trust has consistently been recognised as a crucial ingredient in collaborative practice (Adamson 2011, Stapleton 1998). Sellman (2010) writes that in order to facilitate effective team working, professionals need to trust each other. He found that collaborative working requires professionals to learn new competencies and carry out new roles without rancour and this requires an open, willing and trusting attitude. Adamson (2011) found that trust developed as a result of team members learning to be empathic towards each other, thus demonstrating an ability to fully understand the other member from that person's own perspective. Sellman (2010) suggests that given appropriate conditions, trust in an individual (the 'particular') can develop into trust of their professional group (the 'general'), but points out that conversely, feelings of distrust towards one professional can easily be extended to the whole of their profession.

Trust is more likely to be engendered when each participant feels valued and when relationships are built on mutual respect. Sellman (2006) suggests that trust will only flourish in a climate of trust both amongst individual workers and on an organisational level. The idea of a 'trustworthy' organisation which encourages trust amongst its members (Potter 2002) is essentially a subjective concept but is likely to be absent where the culture is entrenched and defensive with a tendency to blame 'outsiders', where independent thought is not toler-ated, thoughts and feelings are suppressed, leadership is seen as over-control-ling and an all-pervasive anxiety exists (Cruser and Diamond 1996). Another factor impacting on the development of trust is where a partnership arrange-ment is dominated by one particular partner. This can result in tension, distrust and annoyance if the culture of the dominant partner is imposed (Weber and Schweiger 1992 in Glasby and Dickinson 2009). On a macro level, trust will be harder to achieve in an economic and political climate of change and uncer-tainty as this impacts on the ability of the organisation to provide what Bowlby (1969) describes as a sense of a secure base, leading to underlying anxiety and difficulty in establishing trusting relationships.

Personal and Professional Confidence

Confidence is crucial to interprofessional working. Molyneux (2001) found that professionals who were confident in their own role were able to work flexibly across professional boundaries without feeling jealous or threat-ened. However, where personal identity is negative or weak, confidence and assertiveness in an interprofessional context can be adversely affected, compounding a loss of confidence in professional identity. Attacks on per-sonal identity can arise from social divisions associated with, for example, class, gender or ethnicity and can be deeply embedded within the personal-ity. Social differences are inevitably replicated in professional practice (Pollard 2010) and can affect dynamics in teams and have an impact on professional confidence.

Collaborative practice can result in a blurring of roles and knowledge bound-aries and can result in a perception that unique skills are being lost or down-graded (Tucker 2005). This can be experienced as an attack on professional identity and autonomy and seen as part of a process to de-professionalise workers (Miller 2004). Professionals can react with 'discomfort, anxiety and anger' (Frost, Robinson and Anning 2005: 188) as they experience, albeit temporarily, a loss of confidence in their intuitive practice or tacit knowledge and find their level of performance failing to meet their expectations (Eraut 2004). Oliver and Keeping (2010: 101) argue that the 'crisis' precipitated by the permeability of roles associ-ated with interprofessional practice impacts on pre-existing identities and can result in feelings of 'loss, uncertainty, disrespect and marginalization'.

Despite these difficulties, confidence can be reasserted by practitioners if they are able to reconnect with the value base that influenced their original choice of professional role (Hoggett 2005). Oliver and Keeping (2010) suggest that one way of doing this can be to connect with other 'like-minded' individuals, possibly from different professional backgrounds, thus forming a community based on shared values and principles.

Relational skills

Open and honest communication

Communication is one of the most commonly cited competencies needed to work effectively within an interprofessional environment (Cameron, Lart,

Bostock and Coomber 2012, Suter *et al.* 2009) and applies to interactions between professionals and between professionals and service users. It can include skills of negotiation to overcome differences arising from different professional cultures, conflict resolution to tackle disagreements within the team, and skills of conveying information from a uniprofessional perspective, including the ability to adjust the language used rather than using 'in-house' jargon and terminology.

Active listening is another vital tool in facilitating communication and is essential if the knowledge and views of service users are to be recognised and their contribution respected in the pursuit of person-centred care. This is illustrated by the case study in Chapter 4 where Sofie's mother struggles to get her voice heard by professionals. The use of the core conditions of active listening referred to in relation to Sofie's case – namely, respect, empathy and genuineness (Rogers 1980) – involves setting aside stereotypes, preconceived notions and judgements in order to hear what the speaker is saying. It requires the listener to pay close attention to the speaker, to maintain eye contact and to recognise silence as valuable time for the speaker to engage in reflection and thought clarification (Payne 2000). Paraphrasing and summarising can be used to demonstrate understanding and open questions can be used to express interest and encourage further exploration of relevant issues. Payne also identifies the need for critical feedback, combining specific detail, constructive suggestions and encouragement. Open and honest communication is, however, dependent upon a number of previously cited factors including confidence, trust, willingness, openness and respect. As we shall see below, these prerequisites are not always present and can be affected by personal, professional and organisational conditions.

Team working skills

Interprofessional teams succeed when team identity is strong enough to moderate professional identity (Mitchell, Parker and Giles 2011). However, whilst professionals may be based in teams together, this does not necessarily guarantee the formation of a strong team identity or confident team working. As seen above, effective collaboration and effective team working is dependent on positive relationships and good communication. However, as Ward points out, clear communication does not happen by accident and cannot rely solely on bureaucratic channels or meetings. It requires people to 'give of themselves in communication, to receive awkward feedback and to take risks in talking about things which may feel confusing and uncertain at first' (1998: 50). Teams that work well value informal and formal communication which promotes discussion and reflection (Wilson, Ruch, Lymbery and Cooper 2011).

Barriers to interprofessional collaboration

Power

While rarely made explicit, power and status impact significantly on relationships, and have the potential for creating an insidious impact on interprofessional team functioning. Struggles for power are rooted in professional tradition and social difference. Payne identifies power as 'people's capacity to ... get what they want' (2000: 141) exerted through coercion or legitimised through the authority of the profession or organisation. Claims to professional status based upon superior knowledge, autonomy and self-management can result in a reluctance to share power based upon a view that only members of the same profession are in a position to influence decision making, actions and outcomes. Miers (2010) links professional rivalry with the Weberian concept of social closure whereby professional groups strive to protect their status and rewards. In referring to this as the 'professional project', Witz (1992) considered that this closure process results in unhelpfully competitive and conflictual relationships within healthcare, particularly noting the domination of medicine.

The growing dominance of medicalization was noted by Foucault (1973) who wrote about the rising prevalence of the medical model. If power is to be shared or distributed on a basis of the knowledge and expertise of all professionals involved in particular interprofessional initiatives, medical practitioners will need to relinquish traditionally held dominance. Pollard (2010) links medicalization with gender issues in her description of the medicalization of 'normal' physiological and psychological processes. She points out that the feminization of the workplace has failed to make much difference to power and influence within health or social care professions and that both medicalization and unequal gender dynamics influence interprofessional interaction and relationships and act as obstacles to collaborative working between equal partners.

Unequal power distribution can be oppressive (Payne 2000) and can limit participation by service users and professionals alike. A mechanism for recognising the location of power has been identified by Loxley (1997) who poses the set of questions identified in Table 2.1 that are still relevant today. We have supplied examples to illustrate the questions.

─────────── **ACTIVITY** ───────────

Think of an interprofessional initiative with which you have been involved. Using the questions identified by Loxley in Table 2.1, reflect upon the location of power within your chosen initiative.

Power differentials within the interprofessional endeavour often cannot be resolved easily and can lead to envy, resentment and conflict. Different measures can be used to deal with conflict, some less helpful than others. One way is the 'myth of togetherness' (Loxley 1997: 43) whereby team members collude with the status quo and avoid the discomfort of open conflict, a notion also discussed by Warmington, Daniels, Edwards *et al.* (2004). Such avoidance techniques fail to resolve the underlying issues and can result in dysfunctional relationships and constrain creativity and impair efficiency (Drinka and Clark 2000).

As we have seen, power imbalances relate largely to structural issues which may be resistant to change, however, on a team level, certain actions can be taken to prevent or help in the management of conflict. Some examples of useful ground rules can be found below.

- One person talks at a time, while the others listen and don't interrupt
- Commit to establishing a climate of questioning and open discussion
- Everyone has the obligation to give each other honest feedback
- Everyone has an obligation to disagree if they feel they can improve on an intervention
- Recognize that there may be several valid approaches to a situation
- Disagree at the cognitive level versus the affective level
- Create solutions that benefit as many parties as possible

(Drinka and Clark 2000: 160)

QUESTION

- Can you think of any additional ground rules that could help to prevent conflict or enable it to be used creatively?

Table 2.1 Questions to facilitate the location of power within the context of collaborative working

Question	Example
Who defines the problem?	Does everyone make a contribution to problem identification or is this the province of one group?
Whose terms are used?	Is everyone involved able to communicate through the use of mutually agreed and commonly understood terms or does one particular language (professional or service user) predominate?
Who controls the domain or territory?	Is control always mutually negotiated, does it vary in accordance with which professional's knowledge and expertise best fits the particular needs of the service user at a given point in time, or does control sit predominantly with one group?
Who decides upon what resources are needed and how they are allocated?	Are resource issues mutually agreed, determined in accordance with varying professional contributions or dictated by one group?
Who holds whom accountable?	Is it assumed that one group will have overall accountability or is everyone's accountability recognised?
Who prescribes the activity of others?	Is there joint agreement regarding the activities of those involved or does one group prescribe activities?
Who can influence policy makers?	Does one group have a stronger influence than others in lobbying policy makers?

Defences against anxiety

Demands for interprofessional collaboration and other changes to the working environment can cause a great deal of anxiety which often lies beyond the conscious awareness of the individual. In order to protect themselves from this anxiety, individuals can unconsciously enact a defensive process whereby the anxiety is projected into another person. This process can also operate on a group level when individuals hold common anxieties and project their feelings into another group, in so doing strengthening their sense of group membership. Hoggett (2005) suggests this is a crucial process in the maintenance of the identity of the group. Members of other professions are prime targets for such negative projections, and this prepares the ground for a culture of blame to develop.

Hornby and Atkins (2000) point out that the strength of such projections can impede communication and disrupt effective collaboration. Such unhelpful projections need to be withdrawn if professionals are to work collaboratively; however, this entails a disturbance of psychological equilibrium and may be resisted as it means that, once again, the individual must confront and deal with the anxiety they were attempting to avoid. Organisations committed to interprofessional working may therefore find it useful to provide support mechanisms that enable individuals to recognise such psychological defence mechanisms and assist them to find alternative ways of dealing with underlying anxieties.

Strategies to support effective interprofessional working

From the above a number of approaches can be identified as useful in preventing or overcoming some of the difficulties associated with interprofessional working. These are considered below.

Reflection and supervision

A combination of self-reflection and supervision can enable individuals to recognise their strengths and limitations in relation to the knowledge, skills and attitudes required for effective interprofessional working. This mechanism can also be useful in facilitating the recognition of maladaptive defence mechanisms in addition to enabling those involved to identify alternative constructive strategies as a means of coping with threat and uncertainty.

Evaluation

Evaluation can be built into interprofessional working as an integral component of joint working. All involved can engage in group reflection in order to analyse the nature and impact of the interprofessional working relationships. This could include an analysis of the processes involved in decision making, role clarification, negotiation of professional boundaries, work and resource allocation. Group reflection also provides an opportunity for the analysis of power distribution and the strategies used to manage conflict. Group strengths and weaknesses can be identified as a basis for maintaining what works well and negotiating change as and when required.

Learning, education and training

Learning has the potential to change the culture and behaviour of organisations (Deakin Crick, Haigney, Huang *et al.* 2013). Freeth identifies education and training as 'pivotal to providing the conditions and skills required for sustained collaboration' (2001: 40). Bliss, Cowley and White (2000) recommend interprofessional education as a means of enabling professionals to gain an understanding of one another's roles. Interprofessional education could also facilitate learning relating to the ideology of holistic care, recognition of psychological defence mechanisms and conflict management strategies.

Reinforcement of professional identity

Because interprofessional working can involve changes to roles and boundaries, which in turn can erode professional confidence, mechanisms to reinforce a positive professional identity may be useful. Booth and Hewison note that the 'retention of an element of professional uniqueness was necessary to maintain professional confidence' (2002: 39). Reinforcement of allegiance to one's own professional group through attendance at profession-specific meetings may also help to sustain a positive professional identity (Thomas and Spreadbury 2008).

Managerial support

Managerial support can be demonstrated by expressing interest in interprofessional working, acknowledging associated difficulties and investing in time for team building to enable relationships to develop at the commencement of an interprofessional initiative and when new staff replace established members. Clear guidance relating to the parameters within which professionals can negotiate regarding role and resource commitment helps to facilitate devolved responsibility for decision making. Managers also make an important contribution to interprofessional working by selecting appropriate staff, that is, those who have the required authority, experience, enthusiasm, knowledge and skills for effective interprofessional working.

Realistic expectations

Expectations relating to individual and joint outcomes must be realistic otherwise idealised personal or joint goals can result in disappointment and perceptions of failure. Hornby and Atkins (2000) refer to the concept of the *good enough* practitioner as helpful in enabling people to accept that they and others do not necessarily have to achieve perfection. Professional standards do, of course, need to be maintained but participants may have to accept that what is realistically achievable may fall below the level of excellence.

It can be seen from the above that interprofessional working is not necessarily an easy option; however, the problems highlighted in this chapter are not insurmountable. Interprofessional education has been asserted as one approach to enhancing collaboration (Pollard, Miers and Rickaby 2012); however, all professionals involved in health and social care will be involved in interprofessional working at some time and it may not be possible for everyone to access such educational opportunities. Individuals, groups and organisations will therefore benefit from being aware of the processes required for effective interprofessional working, the associated difficulties and strategies which can be utilised to support and enable those involved to optimise their performance in contributing to the interprofessional endeavour.

RECOMMENDED READING

■ Cameron A., Lart R., Bostock L. and Coomber C. (2012) *Research Briefing 41: Factors that Promote and Hinder Joint and Integrated Working between Health and Social Care Services.* London: SCIE.

■ Keeping C. and Barrett G. (2009) Interprofessional practice. In Glasby J. and Dickinson H. (2009) *International Perspectives on Health and Social Care: Partnership Working in Action.* Chichester: Wiley-Blackwell.

■ Pollard K.C., Thomas J. and Miers M. (2010) *Understanding Interprofessional Working in Health and Social Care: Theory and Practice.* Basingstoke: Palgrave Macmillan.

References

Adamson K. (2011) *Interprofessional Empathy in an Acute Healthcare Setting.* Wilfrid Laurier University. http://scholars.wlu.ca. Accessed January 2013.

Axelsson S. and Axelsson R. (2009) From territoriality to altruism in interprofessional collaboration and leadership. *Journal of Interprofessional Care* 23(4): 320–30.

Bliss J., Cowley S. and While A. (2000) Interprofessional working in palliative care in the community: a review of the literature. *Journal of Interprofessional Care* 14: 281–90.

Booth J. and Hewison A. (2002) Role overlap between occupational therapy and physiotherapy during in-patient stroke rehabilitation: an exploratory study. *Journal of Interprofessional Care* 16: 3–40.

Bowlby J. (1969) *Attachment and Loss: Vol. 1. Attachment.* New York: Penguin.

Brown J., Lewis L., Ellis K., Stewart M., Freeman T. and Kasperi M. (2011) Conflict on interprofessional primary health care teams – can it be resolved? *Journal of Interprofessional Care* 25(1): 4–10.

Cameron A. (2011) Impermeable boundaries? Developments in professional and inter-professional practice. *Journal of Interprofessional Care* 25: 53–8.

Cameron A., Lart R., Bostock L. and Coomber C. (2012) *Research Briefing 41: Factors that Promote and Hinder Joint and Integrated Working between Health and Social Care Services.* London: SCIE.

Cruser D.A. and Diamond P.M. (1996) An exploration of social policy and organizational culture in jail-based mental health services. *Administration and Policy in Mental Health* 24:129–48.

Deakin Crick R., Haigney D., Huang S., Coburn T. and Goldspink C. (2013) Learning power in the workplace: the effective lifelong learning inventory and its reliability and validity and implications for learning and development. *The International Journal of Human Resource Management* 24: 2255–72.

Drinka T.J.K. and Clark P.G. (2000) *Health Care Teamwork: Interdisciplinary Practice and Teaching.* Auburn House: Westport.

Foucault M. (1973) *The Birth of the Clinic: Archaeology of Medical Perception.* London: Tavistock.

Freeth D. (2001) Sustaining interprofessional collaboration. *Journal of Interprofessional Care* 15: 37–46.

Frost N., Robinson M. and Anning A. (2005) Social workers in multidisciplinary teams: issues and dilemmas for professional practice. *Child and Family Social Work* 10: 187–96.

Glasby J. and Dickinson H. (2009) *International Perspectives on Health and Social Care: Partnership Working in Action.* Chichester: Wiley-Blackwell.

Hall P. (2005) Interprofessional teamwork: professional cultures as barriers. *Journal of Interprofessional Care* 19(1): 188–96.

Hoggett P. (2005) *Negotiating Ethical Dilemmas in Contested Communities.* ESRC End of Award Report, ref. RES-000-23-0127. www.esrcsocietytoday.ac.uk. Accessed January 2013.

Eraut M. (2004) Learning to change and /or changing to learn. *Learning in Health and Social Care* 3(3): 111–17.

Hornby S. and Atkins J. (2000) *Collaborative Care: Interprofessional, Interagency and Interpersonal* (2nd edn). Oxford: Blackwell Science.

Irvine R., Kerridge I. and Freeman S. (2002) Interprofessionalism and ethics: consensus or clash of cultures? *Journal of Interprofessional Care* 16: 199–210.

Keeping C. and Barrett G. (2009) Interprofessional practice. In Glasby J. and Dickinson H. (2009) *International Perspectives on Health and Social Care: Partnership Working in Action*. Chichester: Wiley-Blackwell, pp. 27–42.

Kvarnstrom S. (2008) Difficulties in collaboration: a critical incident study of interprofessional health care teamwork. *Journal of Interprofessional Care* **22**: 191–203.

Laming, Lord (2003) *Inquiry into the Death of Victoria Climbié*. London: The Stationery Office.

Local Safeguarding Children Board (2009) Serious Case Review – Baby Peter. www.haringeylscb. org. Accessed November 2012.

Loxley A. (1997) *Collaboration in Health and Welfare: Working with Difference*. London: Jessica Kingsley.

McCray J. (2002) Nursing practice in an interprofessional context. In Hogston R. and Simpson P.M. (eds) *Foundations of Nursing Practice: Making the Difference* (2nd edn). Basingstoke: Palgrave Macmillan, pp. 449–69.

Miers M. (2010) Professional boundaries and interprofessional working. In Pollard C., Thomas J. and Miers M. (2010) *Understanding Interprofessional Working in Health and Social Care: Theory and Practice*. Basingstoke: Palgrave Macmillan, pp. 105–21.

Miller C. (2004) *Producing Welfare: A Modern Agenda*. Basingstoke: Palgrave Macmillan.

Mitchell R., Parker V. and Giles M. (2011) When do interprofessional teams succeed? Investigating the moderating roles of team and professional identity in interprofessional effectiveness. *Human Relations* **64**(10): 1321–43.

Molyneux J. (2001) Interprofessional teamworking: what makes teams work well? *Journal of Interprofessional Care* **15**: 29–35.

Nancarrow S. and Borthwick A. (2005) Dynamic professional boundaries in the healthcare workforce. *Sociology of Health and Illness* **27**(7): 897–919.

Oliver B. and Keeping C. (2010) Individual and professional identity. In Pollard C., Thomas J. and Miers M. (eds) *Understanding Interprofessional Working in Health and Social Care: Theory and Practice*. Basingstoke: Palgrave Macmillan, pp. 90–105.

Payne M. (2000) *Teamwork in Multiprofessional Care*. Basingstoke: Macmillan.

Pecukonis E., Doyle O. and Bliss D.L. (2008) Reducing barriers to interprofessional training: promoting interprofessional cultural competence. *Journal of Interprofessional Care* **22**: 417–28.

Pollard K. (2010) The medicalization thesis. In Pollard K., Thomas J. and Miers M. (eds) *Understanding Interprofessional Working in Health and Social Care: Theory and Practice*. Basingstoke: Palgrave Macmillan, pp. 121–38.

Pollard K., Miers M. and Rickaby C. (2012) 'Oh why didn't I take more notice?' Professionals' views and perceptions of pre-qualifying preparation for interprofessional working in practice. *Journal of Interprofessional Care* **26**(5): 355–61.

Pollard C., Thomas J. and Miers M. (2010) *Understanding Interprofessional Working in Health and Social Care: Theory and Practice*. Basingstoke: Palgrave Macmillan.

Potter N.N. (2002) *How Can I Be Trusted? A Virtue Theory of Trustworthiness*. Lanham, MD: Rowman & Littlefield.

Rogers C. (1980) *A Way of Being*. New York: Houghton Mifflin.

Sellman D. (2006) The importance of being trustworthy. *Nursing Ethics* **13**: 105–15.

Sellman D. (2010) Values and ethics in interprofessional working. In Pollard K., Thomas J. and Miers M. (2010) *Understanding Interprofessional Working in Health and Social Care: Theory and Practice*. Basingstoke: Palgrave Macmillan, pp. 156–71.

Sheffield Hallam University (2010) *Interprofessional Capability Framework*. Interprofessional Education Team, Sheffield Hallam University.

Stapleton S.R. (1998) Team-building: making collaborative practice work. *Journal of Nurse-Midwifery* **43**: 12–18.

Suter E., Arndt J., Arthur N., Parboosingh J., Taylor E. and Deutschlander S. (2009) Role understanding and effective communication as core competencies for collaborative practice. *Journal of Interprofessional Care* **23**(1): 41–51.

Thomas J. and Spreadbury K. (2008) Making the best use of opportunities for supervision, learning and development to promote critical best practice. In Jones K., Cooper B. and Ferguson H. (eds) *Best Practice in Social Work: Critical Perspectives*. Basingstoke: Palgrave, pp. 251–65.

Tucker S. (2005) The sum of the parts: exploring youth working identities. In Harrison R. and Wise C. (eds) *Working with Young People*. London: Sage, pp. 204–12.

Ward A. (1998) Helping together. In Ward A. and McMahon L. (eds) *Intuition Is Not Enough: Matching Learning with Practice in Therapeutic Child Care*. London: Routledge, pp. 40–54.

Warmington P., Daniels H., Edwards A., Brown S., Leadbetter J., Martin D. and Middleton D. (2004) *Inter-agency Collaboration: A Review of the Literature*. TLRPIII, University of Birmingham and University of Bath.

Willumsen E., Ahgren B. and Odegard A. (2012) A conceptual framework for assessing interorganizational integration and interprofessional collaboration. *Journal of Interprofessional Care* **26**(3): 198–204.

Wilson K., Ruch G., Lymbery M. and Cooper A. (2011) *Social Work: An Introduction to Contemporary Practice*. Harlow: Pearson Longman.

Witz A. (1992) *Professions and Patriarchy*. London: Routledge.

3

Interprofessional Working with Service Users and Carers

Anne-Laure Donskoy and Katherine C. Pollard

Introduction

The aim of this chapter is to explore the importance of interprofessional working involving service users and carers. We first define terms, identify key pieces of policy and legislation and outline the development of service user and carer involvement in health and social care in the United Kingdom (UK). We then consider how service users and carers negotiate the meaning of inter-professional working; the chapter is mostly written by and presented from the service user perspective. Finally, we discuss the conditions necessary to support service user and carer participation.

Background

Defining terms

The debate about how to refer to people using health or social care services has been well documented (Pollard, Thomas and Miers 2010), yet remains unresolved. The term 'client' is used by some professionals as the indication of an agreement between individuals. Rather than using the term 'patient', which some argue consigns the person to a passive role (Ford 2012), Shaping Our Lives, a leading user-led UK disability organisation, supports the principle of self-identification and considers 'service user' a positive, active term (www.shapingourlives.org.uk).

As one who uses health and social care services, I (A-LD) would argue that each individual should claim which 'identity' they want for themselves; this 'identity' should be shared with and recognised by all relevant professionals. In this chapter, we will refer to individuals who use health and social care services as 'service users'. The term 'carers' will be used to denote individuals who are 'looking after an older relative, a sick friend or a disabled family member' (Carers UK 2011) in an unpaid capacity.

There are two aspects to the involvement of service users and carers in health and social care services. First, it is mandatory for health and social care organisations to include members of the public or patient representatives in commissioning and monitoring local services, as stated in the NHS Act 2006 and the Local Government and Public Involvement in Health Act 2007 (see www.legislation.gov.uk for details of all the Acts referred to in this chapter). Secondly, service users should be able to participate actively in decision making concerning their own care, not only in terms of good practice (Cameron, Lart, Bostock and Coomber 2012, Doel, Carroll, Chambers *et al.* 2007) but also in terms of human rights (UN 2006).

Ideally, the concept of participation should result in empowerment for service users and carers (Thomas 2010). However, as will be discussed below, this is dependent on an appropriate environment being established. Such an environment cannot flourish without active support and contribution from practitioners working together to involve service users.

Key pieces of policy and legislation

Since 2001, UK policies and legislation have stipulated service users' rights to be actively involved in the planning and delivery of care. These include the Health and Social Care Act 2001, Section 11, which mandates more direct forms of service user involvement, as well as the NHS Reform and Healthcare Professionals Act 2002. Subsequently the Health and Social Care Act 2003 established NHS Foundation Trusts; service users and carers can become actively involved in running them. Much of the material in these acts was consolidated through, among others, the NHS Act 2006, the Local Government and Public Involvement in Health Act 2007 and the subsequent Health and Social Care Act 2012.

Concrete examples illustrate the diversity of ways in which legislation has been implemented. For instance, at organisational or structural level, a key national initiative has been the *Expert Patient* programme (DH 2001a), resulting from an overt ambition to develop a 'patient-centred NHS' (DH 2001b). The programme aims to help people living with long-term conditions maintain their personal health and improve their quality of life. It was designed to tap into people's tacit knowledge of their condition and transform it into explicit knowledge, with a view to empowering them and enhancing their relationships with traditional experts (Hardy 2004). However, in other European countries, the concept of 'expert patients' has often taken a different direction, working from an advocacy perspective; for instance in Belgium, 'Experts by Experience' can engage directly with government ministers to negotiate change in services.

Issues of individual rights can also apply to participation. For example, the Mental Capacity Act 2005, together with associated regulations and policies (DH 2010), stipulates that, through the use of specialist advocates and timely, appropriate support, a person has the capacity to make important decisions regarding their care and areas of their lives such as finances and housing. The Act applies not only to persons with mental health issues or learning disabilities, but also to persons with neurological issues (following head trauma, for instance). All professionals involved must adhere to the principles enshrined in the Act.

In the wider international context, the legally binding UN *Convention on the Rights of Persons with Disabilities* (UN 2006), signed and ratified by the UK in 2009, states that persons with disabilities (including mental health issues) have a right to express themselves and to be involved in health and social care services, particularly in relation to their own care. Article 5 makes it clear that denying someone their rights on the basis of disability or incapacity is neither acceptable nor legal under international human rights obligations. Article 12 abolishes the concept of guardianship, whereby someone else makes decisions on the service user's behalf; it was inspired mostly by a striking example from Sweden, the Personal Ombudsman Service (PO-Skåne, undated) which has won international acclaim.

The development of service user and carer participation

The development of legislation to support service user and carer participation in the UK was preceded by the rhetoric of the 1980s and 1990s, which increasingly transformed 'patients' into 'consumers' or 'service users', increasingly viewed as pawns in a financially driven system of managed health (Tritter and McCallum 2006). However, an earlier phase of participation in the UK, before 'patients' became 'service users', occurred through Community Health Councils (CHCs), established in 1974 and abolished in 2003 (Association of Community Health Councils, undated). The Councils' function was to monitor and review NHS services and to recommend improvements, as well as to present patients' views to their local health services. While subsequent bodies failed to meet the increasing need for real representation and influence, the launch of Healthwatch England and of the Healthwatch network (Healthwatch 2013) has raised expectations in terms of genuine representation, scrutiny and leverage. User participation has also always been integral to social care and at the heart of social work values (Doel *et al.* 2007).

Service user and carer participation can be considered analogous with 'citizen participation', as expounded by Arnstein (1969). For a long time her 'ladder of citizen participation' was central to thinking about citizen involvement. The ladder comprises eight levels of increasing participation presented within three categories:

1. Manipulation (Non-participation)
2. Therapy (Non-participation)
3. Informing (Tokenism)
4. Consultation (Tokenism)
5. Placation (Tokenism)
6. Partnership (Citizen Power)
7. Delegated Power (Citizen Power)
8. Citizen Control (Citizen Power).

The ladder still retains some pertinence, in particular when considering how some citizens/service users have little control over their lives. However, it now appears limited with respect to service users and their involvement in health and social care services, because the understanding of participation has evolved greatly over the last forty years.

Building on Arnstein's work, and taking into account the comparative complexity of the current environment, specifically processes and not only outcomes, Tritter (2007) is one of those who have offered other models. He has defined five levels of participation which he claims reflect the subtleties and political demands of that environment more clearly, offering options in the modern 21st century context: participating in decisions about treatment/care; evaluating service provision; planning, designing and commissioning services; teaching; and research.

It must be noted, however, that power (and power sharing) does not automatically 'trickle' down from involvement. All parties need to acknowledge the diversity and complexity of the dynamics of service user involvement. From the point of view of a service user and activist, even Tritter's model remains fairly paternalistic as it fails to acknowledge user-controlled services as genuine alternatives. It also fails to recognise that the success of involvement depends on available support and its manner of implementation. This in turn depends on many other factors, such as the local culture – at profession, team, ward, consultant, speciality, hospital, or local authority level – as much as on resources and infrastructure. For example, it is well known that many professionals' perspectives result from their socialisation during professional education (Reeves, Rice, Conn *et al.* 2009).

ACTIVITY

List all the factors you can think of in a particular environment that may influence how health and/or social care professionals interact with:

1. each other
2. service users/carers.

Participation and interprofessional working

The service user perspective:

> The idea of citizen participation is a little like eating spinach: no one is against it in principle because it is good for you. Participation of the governed in their government is, in theory, the cornerstone of democracy, a revered idea which is vigorously applauded by virtually everyone.
>
> (Arnstein 1969: 216)

Arnstein pointed out that in practice, however, when this principle is advocated by those normally without power, applause is often reduced to 'polite hand claps' because sharing power challenges some fundamental principles and may highlight 'many shades of outright racial, ethnic, ideological and political opposition' (Arnstein 1969: 216). While 1969 may seem like a long time ago, power struggles can still be observed when negotiating meanings, spaces of meaning and expression, or advocacy. Both authors have personally experienced this 'sudden change of tone' when action and meaningful implementation are required (Donskoy 2007).

Service users need clarity in their dealing with health and social care professionals. They want to be listened to, to get clear explanations, to have their questions answered, to share in decisions, and to be treated with respect and empathy (Rose 2003, Wallcraft, Amering, Steffen and Salloum 2012). Negotiating the meaning of interprofessional working from a service user perspective, however, often means dealing with a potentially tentacular beast, where the service user has to juggle different disciplines and perspectives, deal with power differentials and different ways of working, and cope with sometimes impenetrable jargon. Whereas the professionals involved may be tempted to see the service user, who may come with a carer, as yet another case to 'manage', the individual is often just trying to cope with one part of services at a time, learning as they go how best to navigate them.

Service users may be perceived as a homogenous group; this is obviously not the case. In addition to individual preferences and understanding, service users accessing different areas of care often have very different conditions to negotiate. The case of service users who require only physical care is relatively straightforward as, in the UK, they are legally entitled to refuse treatment (DH 2010). Although they may have to assert themselves to combat traditional paternalistic attitudes, their legal and moral right to make decisions about what happens to them is unambiguous. However, mental health care service users can be compulsorily forced to receive treatment without consent, a course of action enshrined in law since the Lunatics Act of 1842 (Fennel 1996). The case of these service users illustrates how they can be constrained by conditions which can be perceived as blackmail, resulting in their being compliant as a means to an end:

> You go to the right groups...you've got to do all that before they let you go, you've got to appear to be keen...because you'll never get out of this place...
>
> (Craik, Bryant, Ryan *et al.* 2010)

This area of care is undoubtedly complex; however, the fact that service users feel they must employ such stratagems in order to have a voice is very far from the ideal of participation. Similarly, the participation of young people in 'community engagement', rather than 'empowering' them, can carry the expectation that they will alter their behaviour to adapt to 'desirable' social norms (Milbourne 2009). For participation to be real and meaningful, members of interprofessional teams may need to challenge their own and each other's assumptions about aspects of practice and care (see, for example, the discussion about the role of the Approved Mental Health Practitioner in Chapter 16).

Whose condition is it anyway?

A crucial aspect of participation concerns the active involvement of service users in decision-making processes relating to their own care. An example of this concerns the introduction of Care Plans into both health and social care, seen as a way of advancing the patient-centred agenda (DWP 2009, Rollins 2011). However, the success of Care Plans varies greatly, depending on the field of health and social care in which they are used. In maternity care, women hold their medical records, something unimaginable in most other areas of care, and totally unthinkable in mental health.

The rhetoric of Care Plans implies that service users and, when applicable, their carers, are involved in both the process and the content of plans. However, in mental health, it is known that Care Plans have not delivered in properly supporting service users at the centre of the process (Donskoy and UFMT 2009). Care Plans have been experienced as a rubber stamping exercise, not happening, happening at the wrong time, not listening to what service users want or need, professionals not attending meetings or leaving them early, meetings not arranged at a suitable time, and so on. Donskoy and colleagues found that:

> Large numbers of service users were still not placed at the centre of the CPA [Care Programme Approach] process: CPA was still a process largely owned by mental health services rather than by the participants in terms of information, process, practicalities and decision-making.
>
> (2009: 110)

The idea of service users at the centre of the process is also about giving them back some control over their condition, something that Illich believed the medical institution dominated excessively:

> By transforming pain, illness, and death from a personal challenge into a technical problem, medical practice expropriates the potential of people to deal with their human condition in an autonomous way and becomes the source of a new kind of un-health.
>
> (2002 [1974]: 919)

The carer perspective

There is increasing recognition that unpaid caring results in considerable savings to services and to tax payers, but also a cost to carers in terms of their own health and well-being. The provision of care within the family is widely reported in most of the literature as 'burdensome' for the caregivers (Chaffey and Fossey 2004, Wane, Larkin, Earl-Gray and Smith 2009). Furthermore, service users and carers are often entwined in a complex relationship that introduces its own challenges into the process of interprofessional working. Carers are sometimes described as barriers to the service user's recovery, either because they lack knowledge about the condition (for a variety of possible reasons), because of their own attitude towards it (particularly in mental health and dementia) or because of over-protectiveness towards the service user (Chaffey and Fossey 2004, Fox 2009, Small, Harrison and Newell 2010, Wane *et al.* 2009). However, due to their intimate knowledge of service users as people living with a condition on an on-going basis, carers have a unique contribution to make which can assist professionals in providing care (Rapaport and Manthorpe 2008). Through the personalisation agenda, the National Carers' Strategy aims to ensure that carers receive appropriate support, including personalised means to access respite care in a variety of forms (Carers Trust 2013).

ACTIVITY

Consider all the issues about a service user's condition and/or lifestyle where they or their carer may have more relevant knowledge than the professionals do.

Supporting service users' and carers' participation in interprofessional working

Practitioners' contribution

Practitioners who cultivate awareness of the need to allow space for service users to express their preferences and to engage actively in decision making about their care can help create situations where genuine participation can occur. When carers are considered as a valid source of knowledge and information, good interprofessional working has the potential of not only alleviating some of the burden carers feel, but also to help smooth the service user–carer relationship itself.

In their study of women carers, Chaffey and Fossey showed that:

> life trajectories and occupations were altered to incorporate caring. The pursuit of their interests, in addition to care-related occupations, appears important for carers to sustain satisfying lives.
>
> (2004: 199)

Practitioners should therefore be aware of carers' needs and may have to offer them support.

It should be clear that every service user is in a unique situation: there is no blanket 'formula' which can be applied to all service users' circumstances. As care is usually provided by an interprofessional team, it is important that *all* team members consider carefully individuals' needs, and be alert to the requirements of their particular situation.

Essential conditions

Within Tritter's (2007) five step model (despite its limitations), interprofessional working has the potential to encompass all aspects of participation. However, participation does not just 'happen'; often it needs negotiation and will only occur if essential elements are encouraged and nurtured. In Chapter 2, Keeping refers to three 'active ingredients' of collaboration, namely 'knowledge', 'attitudes' and 'relational skills' (Suter, Arndt, Arthur *et al.* 2009). In the context of service user involvement in care, it is useful to think about what service users need so they can be actively involved in their own care.

Skilful communication is at the heart of good interprofessional working (Pollard, Rickaby and Miers 2012). Professionals need to relay information consistently between themselves about a person's treatment and care. In theory this happens, but not necessarily in practice (Laming 2009). An essential aspect of communication is listening: unfortunately some staff do not listen to patients or treat them with respect (Donskoy and UFMT 2009, Francis 2013). This behaviour provides evidence for the continued existence of Foucault's concept of 'rupture' which 'increases differences, blurs the lines of communication, and makes it more difficult to pass from one thing to another' (Foucault 1972: 170). Conversely, practising mindful listening has been shown to allow practitioners to be more present in the moment and to hear what service users and carers want to express (Engel, Zarconi, Pethtel and Missimi 2008).

Effective communication, coupled with timely and appropriate information, can enable individuals to make meaningful decisions. Service users require clarity about, for instance, the side effects and limitations of particular treatments. They may also at times need independent advice. Professionals should be able to help them, possibly through Patient Decision Aids which are designed to help patients make difficult decisions when there is no clinical evidence to suggest that one treatment/test option is better than another.

In some areas of health and social care, for example mental health, a person's lack of mental capacity or insight is often cited as the reason for not involving them in decision-making about their care (Lloyd and King 2003). However, as mentioned above, the Mental Capacity Act 2005 demands that professionals should support individuals to make their own choices. It is the responsibility of team professionals to ensure that appropriate and timely information is offered to service users that will help empower them to make the right choices for themselves (DH 2012, NICE 2011).

Simply giving someone a leaflet, or signposting them to a telephone number or a website, does not constitute provision of appropriate information. The person may need support, for instance, in accessing information in a specific format or language (Ásmundsdóttir 2009). The issue of health literacy is critical as it enables a person to read, understand, evaluate and use health information to make appropriate decisions about their own health and the care that they receive (Nutbeam 2000). Conversely, low health literacy is associated with health inequalities and increased levels of hospitalisation, as it is often accompanied by low ability to access and understand information and to make appropriate decisions (Coulter, Parsons and Askham 2008, Nutbeam 2000). Where information is written in complex language and may require deciphering, professionals should check with service users whether or not they require support; this needs to be done in a simple, non-patronising way as many people may feel unable to ask for such help. It is obviously important to allow time for someone to understand information and to reflect on decisions that have been or will be made.

Power issues are central to the concept of service user involvement in interprofessional working. These are about respect and creating the necessary space for all relevant processes to take place (see Chapter 2 for more detail). When conditions are right, the balance of power can shift in favour of a more flexible dynamic between service users (and carers) and professionals, allowing service users to put their point of view across more assertively (Goffman 1961, Kleinman 1988).

Language use is associated with power issues, and can result in power being shifted towards medical and other professionals. A particular problem involves service users being excluded from participation due to the impenetrability of clinicians' language (Hardy 2004). Other problems occur when language is used to confer identity on service users. For example, the use of the word 'girls' to refer to women using the maternity services effectively infantilises them, supporting a discourse surrounding the control of birth which implies that they cannot legitimately challenge the power of healthcare professionals (the 'adults' in this situation) (Pollard 2007).

Mental health service users have used language to (re)gain control over their destiny as patients and citizens. For instance, they have been using the expression 'survivor' to describe their experiences, 'because we have *survived* [italics added] an ostensibly helping system which places major obstacles across our path to self-determination' (Campbell 1992: 117, cited in Cresswell 2005). The term itself reveals a dynamic political function which aims to change self and societal conceptions of mental health service users. It highlights human activism, a counterpoint to the experts' power to control the language of definition and the importance of narrative transformation. The main concept here is self-determination as a means of recovering agency and self-hood. Health care professionals must acknowledge users as persons with agency and not passive subjects of their conditions or of the health care system. Members of interprofessional teams need to discuss these issues with service users and with each other.

Engaging in good interprofessional working which empowers service users and carers demands that health and social care practitioners employ high-level skills, which unfortunately, not all possess (Pollard 2008). Well-designed training courses can improve the communication skills of the health and social care staff, for example, their use of 'mindful listening' (Engel *et al.* 2008), and their awareness of relevant issues, for example, the appropriate use of language.

ACTIVITY

Consider how staff in your area of practice could be supported in order to engage in genuine interprofessional working with service users and carers. Think about both organisational and personal factors.

Conclusion

The involvement of service users and carers in interprofessional working is not new, but has evolved and become more complex over the last decade. As professionals gain more high level engagement skills and new legislation influences both awareness and practice, professionals should be moving away from traditionally paternalistic perspectives. The practitioner's aim should be to achieve the right balance between offering individuals support and advice, and respecting their right to self-determination. Conversely, as service users and carers become more involved in making decisions about their own care, their knowledge improves and they are better able to negotiate the complexities of health and social care services. Suitable training can support practitioners to engage in essential cooperation with service users and carers, to create the conditions needed for interprofessional working which can result in a genuinely user-centred service.

━━━━━━━━━━━━━━━━━━ **RECOMMENDED READING** ━━━━━━━━━━━━━━━━━━

■ Coulter A. (2011) *Engaging Patients in Healthcare*. Maidenhead: Open University Press.

■ McPhail M. (2007) *Service User and Carer Involvement: Beyond Good Intentions*. Edinburgh: Dunedin Academic Press.

■ Staniszewska S. and Denegri S. (2013) Patient and public involvement in research: future challenges. *Evidence-Based Nursing* **16**(3): 69.

■ Wallcraft J., Schrank B. and Amering M. (eds) (2009) *Handbook of Service User Involvement in Mental Health Research*. Oxford: John Wiley & Sons.

References

Arnstein S. (1969) A ladder of citizen participation in the USA. *Journal of the American Institute of Planners* 35(4): 216–24.

Ásmundsdóttir E.E. (2009) Creation of new services: collaboration between mental health consumers and occupational therapists. *Occupational Therapy in Mental Health* 25: 115–26.

Association of Community Health Councils (undated) The golden age of patient and public involvement. www.achcew.org.uk. Accessed August 2013.

Cameron A., Lart R., Bostock L. and Coomber C. (2012) *Research Briefing 41: Factors that Promote and Hinder Joint and Integrated Working between Health and Social Care Services*. London: SCIE.

Carers Trust (2013) *National Carers Strategy*. www.professionals.carers.org. Accessed June 2013.

Carers UK (2011) *Carers UK: The Voice of Carers*. www.carersuk.org. Accessed February 2012.

Chaffey L. and Fossey E. (2004) Caring and daily life: occupational experiences of women living with sons diagnosed with schizophrenia. *Australian Occupational Therapy Journal* 51: 199–207.

Coulter A., Parsons S. and Askham J. (2008) Where are the patients in decision-making about their own care? Paper presented at the WHO European Ministerial Conference on Health Systems, Tallinn, Estonia.

Craik C., Bryant W., Ryan A., Barclay S., Brooke N., Mason A. and Peter R. (2010) A qualitative study of service user experiences of occupation in forensic mental health. *Australian Occupational Therapy Journal* 57: 539–44.

Cresswell M. (2005) Psychiatric survivors and testimonies of self-harm. *Social Science and Medicine* 61: 1668–77.

DH (Department of Health) (2001a) *The Expert Patient: A New Approach to Chronic Disease Management for the 21st Century*. London: DH.

DH (2001b) *Shifting the Balance of Power within the NHS: Securing Delivery*. London: DH.

DH (2010) *The Mental Capacity Act 2005*. http://webarchive.nationalarchives.gov.uk. Accessed February 2012.

DH (2012) *The NHS Constitution for England*. London: DH.

Doel M., Carroll C., Chambers E., Cooke J., Hollows A., Laurie L. and Nancarrow S. (2007) Developing measures for effective service user and carer participation. *Stakeholder Participation*. London: SCIE.

Donskoy A.-L. (2007) La Participation Usagere: Oser, Oser. *Confluences* 46–7.

Donskoy A.-L. and UFMT (User Focused Monitoring Team) (2009) *The Experiences of the Care Programme Approach in Bristol: How Socially Inclusive Is It?* Bristol: Bristol Mind.

DWP (Department for Work and Pensions) (2009) *Care Programme Approach (CPA)*. www.dwp. gov.uk. Accessed February 2012.

Engel J.D., Zarconi J., Pethtel L.L. and Missimi S.A. (2008) *Narrative in Health Care*. Oxford: Radcliffe.

Fennel P. (1996) *Treatment without Consent: Law, Psychiatry and the Treatment of Mentally Disordered People since 1845*. London: Routledge.

Ford, S. (2012) *Patients assume passive role to avoid 'difficult' label*. www.nursingtimes.net. Accessed January 2013.

Foucault M. (1972) *The Archaeology of Knowledge*. London: Tavistock.

Fox J. (2009) A participatory action research project evaluating a carers' representation group – Carers Against Stigma. *Mental Health Review Journal* **14**(4): 25–35.

Francis R. (2013) *Final Report of the Independent Inquiry into Care Provided by Mid Staffordshire NHS Foundation Trust*. www.midstaffsinquiry.com. Accessed June 2013.

Goffman E. (1961) *Asylums: Essays on the Social Situation of Mental Patients and other Inmates*. London: Penguin.

Hardy P. (2004) *The Expert Patient Programme: A Critical Review*. www.pilgrimprojects.co.uk. Accessed February 2012.

Healthwatch (2013) Healthwatch: your spotlight on health and social care services. www.health-watch.co.uk. Accessed August 2013.

Illich I. (2002 [1974]) Medical nemesis. *British Medical Journal* **57**(12): 919–22.

Kleinman A. (1988) *The Illness Narratives: Suffering, Healing, and the Human Condition*. New York: Basic Books.

Laming, Lord (2009) *The Protection of Children in England: A Progress Report*. Norwich: The Stationery Office.

Lloyd C. and King R. (2003) Consumer and carer participation in mental health services. *Australasian Psychiatry* **11**(2): 180–4.

Milbourne L. (2009) Valuing difference or securing compliance? Working to involve young people in community settings. *Children and Society* **23**: 347–63.

NICE (National Institute for Health and Clinical Excellence) (2011) Service user experience in adult mental health: improving the experience of care for people using adult NHS mental health services. www.nice.org.uk. Accessed June 2013.

Nutbeam D. (2000) Health literacy as a public health goal: a challenge for contemporary health education and communication strategies into the 21st century. *Health Promotion International* **15**(3): 259–67.

PO-Skåne (undated) *Swedish user-run service with Personal Ombud (PO) for psychiatric patients*. www.po-skane.org. Accessed January 2012.

Pollard K.C. (2007) Discourses of unity and division: an exploration of interprofessional working among midwives in an English NHS maternity unit. PhD thesis. Bristol: University of the West of England.

Pollard K.C. (2008) Non-formal learning and interprofessional collaboration in health and social care: the influence of the quality of staff interaction on student learning about collaborative behaviour in practice placements. *Learning in Health and Social Care* **17**(1): 12–26.

Pollard K.C., Rickaby C. and Miers M. (2012) 'Oh why didn't I take more notice?' Professionals' views and perceptions of pre-qualifying preparation for interprofessional working in practice. *Journal of Interprofessional Care* **26**(5): 355-61.

Pollard K.C., Thomas J. and Miers M. (eds) (2010) *Understanding Interprofessional Working in Health and Social Care: Theory and Practice*. Basingstoke: Palgrave Macmillan.

Rapaport J. and Manthorpe J. (2008) Family matters: developments concerning the role of the nearest relative and social worker under mental health law in England and Wales. *British Journal of Social Work* **38**: 1115–31.

Reeves S., Rice K., Conn L.G., Miller K.-L., Kenaszchuk C. and Zwarenstein M. (2009) Interprofessional interaction, negotiation and non-negotiation on general internal medicine wards. *Journal of Interprofessional Care* **23**(6): 633–45.

Rollins H. (2011) Practical care: how to improve care plans. *Nursing and Residential Care* **13**(11): 541–3.

Rose D. (2003) Partnership, co-ordination of care and the place of user involvement. *Journal of Mental Health* **12**: 59–70.

Shaping Our Lives (undated) *Definitions.* www.shapingourlives.org.uk. Accessed January 2012.

Small N., Harrison J. and Newell R. (2010) Carer burden in schizophrenia: considerations for nursing practice. *Mental Health Practice* **14:** 21–5.

Suter E., Arndt J., Arthur N., Parboosingh J., Taylor E., and Deutschlander S. (2009) Role understanding and effective communication as core competencies for collaborative practice. *Journal of Interprofessional Care* **23**(1): 41–51.

Thomas J. (2010) Service users, carers and issues for collaborative practice. In Pollard K.C. Thomas J. and Miers M. (eds) *Understanding Interprofessional Working in Health and Social Care: Theory and Practice.* Basingstoke: Palgrave Macmillan, pp. 171–85.

Tritter J. (2007) *Where Next for User Involvement?* Bristol: University of the West of England.

Tritter J.Q. and McCallum A. (2006) The snakes and ladders of user involvement: moving beyond Arnstein. *Health Policy* **76**: 156–8.

UN (United Nations) (2006) *UN Convention on the Rights of Persons with Disabilities. www.un. org. Accessed June 2013.*

Wallcraft J., Amering M., Steffen S. and Salloum I.M. (2012). Evaluators and assessment process in person-centred integrative diagnosis. *The International Journal of Person Centered Medicine* **2**: 201–4.

Wane J., Larkin M., Earl-Gray M. and Smith H. (2009) Understanding the impact of an Assertive Outreach Team on couples caring for adult children with psychosis. *Journal of Family Therapy* **31**: 284–309.

PART II

Professional Perspectives

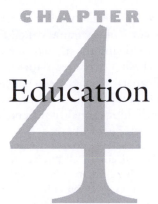

Education

Jane Tarr

Introduction

This chapter provides an overview of educational provision for children and young people outlining opportunities for collaborative practice and enhanced communication between staff in schools and other public service agencies. Inclusive education involves learners who require additional support to enhance their learning capacity. If coherent provision is to be achieved communication processes between professionals across different agencies must be effective. The case study of a child with profound hearing loss is used to illustrate the importance of effective communication skills within and between public service agencies for children within the compulsory education system.

Education services

The education service in England and Wales provides compulsory education for all children from the age of five. The Education and Skills Act 2008 (www.legislation.gov.uk) requires young people in England to participate in education or training to the age of 17 from 2013 and to the age of 18 from 2015. By law parents must send their child to school unless granted special dispensation for home education. Compulsory education usually lasts for seven years in primary and seven years in secondary school although some counties have middle schools for 9- to 13-year-olds. All 3- and 4-year-olds are entitled to 15 hours of free nursery education for 38 weeks a year, until compulsory school begins.

Schools and teachers have responsibility for the learning of children and young people within a common curriculum framework (Table 4.1). The demise of local education authorities following the merger of education and social services provision in the Children Act 2004 (www.legislation.gov.uk) also permits schools to take responsibility for financial management which has implications for how educationalists engage with other public services, particularly in providing for learners who have additional educational requirements. The revised standards for September 2012 expect teachers to have:

> a clear understanding of the needs of all pupils, including those with special educational needs; those of high ability; those with English as an additional language; those with disabilities; and be able to use and evaluate distinctive teaching approaches to engage and support them
>
> (TA 2011: 1)

and to:

> develop effective professional relationships with colleagues, knowing how and when to draw on advice and specialist support; deploy support staff effectively…communicate effectively with parents with regard to pupils' achievements and well-being.
>
> (TA 2011: 1)

If a child has a difficulty in learning greater than most learners in a school, that child may be recognised as having special educational needs (SEN) and may require differentiated teaching and learning approaches to meet her or his educational needs. If a broad range of children's services is required, a statement of

Table 4.1   Educational provision in the UK

Age	Provision	Document
Birth –5	15 hours nursery provision for all from 3 years old	**Early Years Foundation Stage 0–5years (DfE 2012a)** • quality and consistency in all early years settings, so that every child makes good progress and no child gets left behind; • a secure foundation through learning and development opportunities which are planned around the needs and interests of each individual child and are assessed and reviewed regularly; • partnership working between practitioners and with parents and/ or carers; • equality of opportunity and anti-discriminatory practice, ensuring that every child is included and supported.
5–7 7–11 11–14 14–16	Compulsory education for all	At the time of writing the National Curriculum for primary schools is being reviewed to give greater freedom to teachers to respond to the needs of the learners in their schools.
16–18	Changing to become compulsory	At the time of writing the curriculum for secondary schools and further education colleges is being reviewed to enable greater level of flexibility for schools, teachers, and learners

special educational needs to clarify the additional support required is compiled (DfES 2001). The move towards inclusive education requires teachers to work collaboratively to meet children's educational needs. Following the *SEN Green Paper Consultation* (DfE 2011), 20 Pathfinders involving 31 local authorities and their health partners began to explore proposals for a single assessment process for 0- to 25-year-olds, personal budgeting, the role of parents, and the practice of multiagency working. This system may increase responsibility for those working closest to learners, thus potentially reduce regional collective provision. A March 2013 report indicates that progress has been made with multiagency working between education, health and social services with high levels of family engagement and that some authorities are setting up joint commissioning approaches (DfE/DH 2013).

School context

Children in primary schools spend most of each year with one class teacher. Adapting to many different teachers (each responsible for a specific curriculum area) can be challenging for learners as they transition, at age 11, to secondary school. In school pupils interact with teachers and a headteacher, administrative staff, school meals supervisory assistants, cleaners, and caretakers. In the classroom they might meet trained nursery nurses (during early years), unqualified teaching assistants (who support teachers), and learning support assistants and learning mentors (who support learners). Within the wider school they may meet health practitioners (for example, school nurses, and speech and language therapists), and social care practitioners. Time for effective liaison and communication between any additional adults and teacher, and between different teachers, is crucial if interventions in children's learning are to be successful, particularly for those pupils identified as having special educational needs.

Education and social services came together as the Children and Young People's Service following the Children Act 2004 which states that all different agencies involved with children have a duty to cooperate to ensure the well-being of children and young people in relation to:

(a) physical and mental health and emotional well-being;
(b) protection from harm and neglect;
(c) education, training and recreation;
(d) the contribution made by them to society;
(e) social and economic well-being.

(Children Act 2004, Part 2, section 10)

Staff in schools are valued colleagues and may be the first to notice if a child is experiencing harm and/or neglect. A specific teacher holds responsibility for child protection in every school and holds the duty to cooperate with colleagues in social services, police, and health, if concerns are raised. The revised version of *Working Together to Safeguard Children* (DfE 2013a) emphasises that all professionals hold responsibility for safeguarding children and that health practitioners, social workers, police, schools and other voluntary or community organisations need to work together. (Further information about this aspect of interprofessional practice can be found in Chapters 11 and 14.)

While financial constraint has reduced the range of professionals working within Children and Young People's Services, local authorities continue to employ some of the following: administrators, education resource managers, advisory staff, curriculum support teachers, children's officers, education welfare officers, educational psychologists, behaviour support teachers/assistants, special needs teachers/assistants, ethnic minority achievement teachers, early years and childcare educationalists, hospital teachers, and community education officers, as well as social workers and a range of social care workers. At the time of writing, key personnel available to support learners with additional requirements include the professionals outlined in the following paragraphs.

Educational psychologists have a doctorate in educational psychology and experience of professional work with children. They work within a team to support schools, families and children, assisting teachers in devising strategies and activities for individual children, groups of children, classes or the whole school. Such work may include specific individual assessments, presentations, the introduction of behaviour support programmes, leading discussions on teaching and learning approaches, and allocating additional monies to employ, for example, learning support assistants or counsellors (DfEE 2000a). The educational psychologist often oversees compilation of statements of educational need (DfES 2001). Following the *Every Child Matters* (DCSF 2004) agenda, Farrell, Woods, Lewis *et al.* (2006) clarified that educational psychologists would engage with multiagency and school work related to early years education at four levels: the individual child; groups of children; the school; and the local authority.

The education welfare officer (or education social worker) works closely with families to ensure access to educational provision and with schools to ensure children and young people feel confident to attend school. They liaise with social services when similar goals for child and family are shared by community care workers and social workers.

The special needs support service (SNSS) may consist of advisors, teachers and assistants with expertise in teaching and learning for pupils with special needs. The SNSS advisor supports schools in developing systems, policies and teaching approaches to enhance a school's capacity to include special educational needs pupils. The SNSS advisor also gets involved in compiling statements of educational need and in allocating resources. Teachers and assistants work alongside teachers to enhance children's learning capacity while the behaviour support team help to address issues of pupil behaviour.

Early years

The Sure Start initiative (DfEE 2000b) encouraged collaboration between social, education, and health services to support families with children under compulsory school age to access their 15 hours of free nursery provision. Funding through Sure Start has ceased but Children's Centres continue to develop where children's services come together to provide for families under the same roof. Recent reviews of Sure Start children's centre guidance indicates that they are 'hubs for multi-agency teams' (DfE 2013b: 19) and encourage interprofessional practice while holding a strong emphasis on family involvement. When nursery provision is unsuitable, access may be available to a Portage educational programme delivered in the child's home by a tutor working alongside parents to provide activities promoting child development. Early years provision depends upon individual local authorities and voluntary bodies, and it is often difficult for families to know what is available. The merger of education and social services encourages sharing of knowledge and information between professionals and with families.

Compulsory schooling

The transition from small-scale nursery to compulsory education can be traumatic for children and families. Family centres encourage working partnerships between professionals from different agencies to offer personal support when compulsory schooling begins. Interagency cooperation becomes crucial as education becomes a major provider for children and families who are socially disadvantaged or whose children require additional health or educational support (Edwards 2009). In the UK, the Children and Families Bill 2013 demonstrates the value of supporting families from a range of services.

The Children and Families Bill 2013 also proposes revisions to the *Special Educational Needs Code of Practice* (DfES 2001). Updates include developing a system that supports children and young people 'from birth to age 25; raising aspirations; putting children, young people and parents at the centre of decisions; and giving them greater choice and control over their support so that they can achieve at school and college and make a successful transition to adult life' (DfE 2013c: 15).

The 2001 *Special Educational Needs Code of Practice* provides guidance for parents, educationalists and other professionals to support children who find learning difficult. The Special Educational Needs and Disability Act (SENDA) 2001 (www.legislation.gov.uk) established legal rights for disabled students to be included in pre- and post-16 education. This was supported further by the Disability Discrimination Act 2005 (www.legislation.gov.uk) which encourages deeper levels of inclusion in mainstream schools and was included within the Equality Act 2010 (www.legislation.gov.uk) to provide families with rights of participation in decision making regarding their child's education. The next steps build upon this legislation to enable families to have more choice; moreover the expectation for different agencies to cooperate and work collaboratively remains highly valued.

With the support of the special education needs coordinator, the class teacher devises teaching strategies, individual education plans with specific targets for the child, and effective review and monitoring systems. Where the needs of the child cannot be met within existing resources, the school will seek support from School Action Plus (DfES 2001). This official recognition of external agencies' involvement could include consultation with: the educational psychologist or special needs support team; the speech and language therapist or physiotherapist within the health service; or the social worker or community care worker within social services.

Inclusive education means mainstream schools will admit children with learning difficulties requiring teachers to work interprofessionally. A case study was chosen from a larger study (Tarr 2003) involving interviews with 12 parents and 12 different professionals which found that effective communication had a major influence on a positive experience for children and their families. Six aspects were identified for consideration as follows:

a) active listening skills
b) conversational competence
c) different modes of communication
d) sharing of knowledge and information
e) building effective professional relationships
f) building, using and maintaining professional networks.

(Tarr 2003: 210)

The following case study, concerning a child with profound hearing impairment, offers insight into the need for effective communication between all professionals involved with the child and family. Through reflection upon the experiences outlined in the study each of the six aspects of communication are explored and questions posed for the reader. It is intended that the reader can reflect upon their own experiences and enhance interprofessional working practice for the best interests of the child and their family. Names have been changed to ensure anonymity.

CASE STUDY: Sofie

Sofie, an 11-year-old white girl, was born with bilateral centro-neuro hearing loss. An only child, living with her mother and stepfather, she attends a special school for the hearing impaired where instruction is in British Sign Language. Her mother discovered through trial and error that signing was valuable for Sofie and after a long battle with her then oralist local authority, moved house to find a school with signing as the medium of instruction. The family has extensive interaction with the health service particularly with the paediatrician, ear nose and throat consultant, and general practitioner. Communication within the education service has included mainstream schoolteachers, peripatetic teachers of the deaf, a learning support assistant, a special needs support teacher, an educational psychologist and special educational needs advisors. Sofie has attended a mainstream school with additional support, a specialised unit attached to a mainstream school and a special school for the hearing impaired. The family receives disability carer's allowance but does not have a social worker. They have received support from council housing departments who on three occasions have housed them near to their chosen school. Sofie's mother belongs to the National Deaf Children's Society and is secretary for the local deaf association which runs a centre for the deaf. She is also a school meals supervisor and an active parent governor at Sofie's school.

a) Active listening skills

Unlike the peripatetic teachers for the deaf in this location and time, Sofie's mother understood that hearing aids offered no benefit to Sofie's profound hearing loss and that Sofie could only communicate through sign language. In contrast, her local authority suggested an oralist approach seeking to amplify residual hearing with hearing aids and encourage lip reading. If the professionals had adopted Rogers' (1980) *open listening* approach for Sofie's mother, showing respect, empathy and genuineness, they could have incorporated her knowledge and provided more appropriately targeted support for the family.

CASE STUDY continued

Sofie's mother says: 'When Sofie was eight months we went for the statutory hearing tests, the spoon in a cup and rattle; she happened to move her arm so she passed that, I totally and strongly disagreed. I decided to seek a second opinion and went to the University where they did a test with electrodes, they said she had a severe hearing loss. We went back to the hospital again because it turned out that the professionals doing the machinery had not done it well, only to be told that she was definitely profoundly deaf with bilateral central-neuro hearing loss. So all of a sudden I had all these wonderful professionals with years of experience coming into my home and my life telling me what to do. I had two peripatetic teachers for the deaf who told me that if Sofie signed and went into sign language, which wasn't really necessary these days because hearing aids are marvellous, she would never read, never write and go to a boarding school at five.'

This illustrates the importance of listening, and of acknowledging different perspectives in pursuit of shared problem-solving (DfES 2001). Developing active listening skills to recognise potential conflict within different viewpoints can assist incorporation of divergent thinking when devising innovative responses to challenging situations. An approach to Sofie's profound hearing impairment involving active listening, would recognise the knowledge and views of both mother and practitioners enabling different approaches to be explored in Sofie's best interest.

QUESTIONS

- What are the implications of actively listening to clients' viewpoints?
- What might you learn from listening to the perspective of another professional within your area of practice?
- Give an example of where conflicting viewpoints may occur in your area of practice.

CASE STUDY continued

'The ear nose and throat consultant at the hospital asked me how it was going and I told him I had started signing and he told me it wasn't a proper language. I asked him if he signed and he ignored me so I shouted again and he said, "I do not need to because I can hear" my response was to say "Aren't you lucky" picked up my kid and walked out and never spoke another word to him ... I am angry because if the professionals in the field of deafness had explained that they did not accept the place of signing I would have moved when she was a toddler to somewhere appropriate. I knew little about how counties thought differently about deaf community' (Sofie's mother).

'They keep mothers or parents in total ignorance of what is available for the child, what can be done, what cannot be done. Eventually we learned that county policy was not to consider using a signed approach until the child was six or seven years old. So Sofie was refused access to communication. If that had happened to a hearing child for six years, can you imagine what social services would do to you but you have a deaf child and they support it' (Sofie's stepfather).

---

b) Conversational competence

The words of Sofie's mother and stepfather illustrate difficulties facing professionals in conversations of potential conflict. Explaining reasons for county available provision required high levels of conversational competence involving linguistic skill and sensitivity to others' language use. Clients appreciate a professional's ability to 'participate in conversation situations and to debate or persuade' (Svensson 1990: 53) yet few public service professionals have time to engage in such conversation even though the capacity to converse, persuade and convince is accepted as valuable in building effective interprofessional understanding (Svensson 1990).

Conflicting communication strategies for the hearing impaired had a detrimental impact upon Sofie's family. Communication might have been enhanced had the consultant explained his views about signing, and listened to the views of the mother. In this context sensitive linguistic skill can minimise complex disciplinary specific language and encourage well-informed exchanges of perspective. Sofie's mother found the most useful conversations involved informal exchanges such as those between parent and learning support assistant, and with regularly visiting family friends. Recognising that context has an impact upon conversational outcomes may result in more suitable venues for interaction. A family centre for those with young children is an ideal opportunity for professionals to interact informally with both clients and professionals from different agencies.

QUESTIONS

■ Consider areas in your professional conversations where misconceptions can arise for the lay person.

■ Identify some informal contexts where conversation between different professionals might take place.

c) Different modes of communication

Professionals communicate in writing, by telephone and in face-to-face interactions during formal or informal meetings. Interprofessional practice may require a range of communicative strategies although electronic modes are fast becoming the norm. The multiple understandings that abound in interprofessional collaboration may lead institutions to create what Young (2000) describes as *inclusive political communication systems* through a variety of modes. Leaflets and brochures are frequently used to provide information about professional services but the language of such texts can be inaccessible and may deter parents from pursuing additional financial support.

CASE STUDY continued

To ensure Sofie received additional resources, a statement of her special educational needs was compiled following a multidisciplinary assessment involving Sofie's parents as well as professionals from health and education services. The outcome listed the nature of the additional support to be allocated. The contribution from mother in regard to Sofie's signing ability was only included on her insistence although she objected to it being couched as *mother says;* as if it was not to be taken seriously. Sofie's mother continues: 'So I rang up to ask. I kept ringing, I did not care what else was going on. Tell her I am in a meeting you could hear it all. I kept ringing, I did not care if I was a nuisance, at the end of the day my focus is my child. I cannot worry about what else they are dealing with.'

Sofie received full-time support from Sally, a learning support assistant. Sofie's mother explains: 'Sally was good, the support of £500 came our way, so we hired a video recorder and we did the Oxford Reading Tree. So we used to go round her house and we videoed in sign all these books, sometimes the shortened versions so we could give her access in her language, to help her to learn English grammar. It was working, she read well.'

Communication often proceeds in institutionalised, taken-for-granted forms within professional groups. The statement of educational needs to which parents are asked to contribute is written in formal language. Sofie's mother's contribution was not taken seriously. She used the telephone when trying to gain a place for Sofie in a new school. With the help of the learning support assistant, she created signed videos of Sofie's reading books.

Reflection on different modes of communication leads to the recognition that there are stereotypical expectations in relation to people's understanding of different *languages*. Language is 'embedded in the shapes and characters of our abiding social institutional forms' (Vass 1991: 223) and cannot easily be redistributed without considerable change. Professionals may need to consider enhancing unfamiliar modes of communication in order to ensure understanding across disciplines.

QUESTIONS

■ List the range of ways in which you communicate with clients.

■ Consider the most successful modes of communication in your professional work.

■ How might you enhance communication systems between different professionals?

CASE STUDY continued

Sofie's mother maintains connections with the deaf community stating: 'Our social life is either with the deaf or nothing.' After moving across the country she joined the deaf centre, the deaf youth club, became a parent governor at her child's school and joined the policy committee for the school's family centre for deaf children. As she says 'I stuck my nose in everywhere, picked up every bit of paper going to know what is the difference between total communication, bilingualism and a signing unit.'

Following the initial limited resource allocation, Sofie's mother sought advice from the National Deaf Children's Society and managed to obtain full-time signing support for Sofie during school time. She realised that the debate was complex but that she needed to be insistent if her child was going to get appropriate provision.

---

d) Sharing knowledge and information

Parents often know more about their child than a professional with responsibility for many children, something not always appreciated by professionals. Interactions within the deaf community provided information for the family while voluntary bodies were supportive in ensuring knowledge was shared with Sofie's parents. This suggests it might be beneficial for professionals to cultivate relationships with voluntary organisations to gain insight into different perspectives.

Sharing knowledge and information depends upon individuals having time to interact. Building partnerships through joint planning of provision for vulnerable children is developing and professionals involved in such partnerships should anticipate sharing knowledge. The *SEND Green Paper* (2012) which leads into the Children and Families Bill 2013 states that 'we want to make it easier for professionals and services to work together, and we want to create the conditions that encourage innovative and collaborative ways of providing better support for children, young people and families' (DfE 2012b: 66). Successful sharing between professions and agencies requires both the ability to communicate complex knowledge in simple terms and the determination to avoid jargon and disciplinary-specific language. Sharing of knowledge can lead to joint problem solving, challenging assumptions and ideologies, and result in innovative outcomes.

Professionals engaged in sharing knowledge and information must be sensitive to protecting client confidentiality, particularly when working in child protection where ethical concerns of confidentiality between agencies can be problematic (DfE 2013). Keeping parents informed can alleviate some of the difficulty. Sofie's mother realised when Sofie started school that information had not been shared between health and education. Consequently the teachers were inadequately prepared to support her in mainstream school.

The *Special Educational Needs Code of Practice* (DfES 2001) promotes parent partnership schemes within, but independent of, each local authority with the aim of supporting families with children with special educational needs. Sofie's mother was unhappy with the statement of educational need, which awarded part-time support from a signing support assistant. As she put it 'I said I thought she had to attend school full time? They said she does. I said she couldn't with only 17.5 hours support she will only be there for 17.5 hours so when do I bring her in and when do I take her home?' With help from the National Deaf Children's Society, *mother says* was removed from the document and full-time signing support was awarded.

With help from voluntary bodies Sofie's family moved twice to ensure a place in school. Had the health and education services shared information with housing departments the family may have been better supported. The creation of systemic procedures for interprofessional sharing of knowledge and information developed through jointly planned and jointly funded projects can lead to what Roaf (2002) calls *joined up action*.

QUESTIONS

- What knowledge/information can parents access in deciding which school to send their child?
- What further knowledge might be shared between health and education services at the start of compulsory schooling?
- How might you explain your knowledge of a particular child's needs to a professional working in another discipline?

e) Building effective professional relationships

Building professional relationships requires resources and time. The example below outlines how relationships between school and family can break down. Building interprofessional relationships based upon mutual respect and cooperation requires structural change. Interprofessional review meetings aim for the best solution for a child but may not encourage open discussion of issues in the absence of the trust condition of interprofessional working (Sellman 2010).

CASE STUDY continued

Sofie's mother explains: 'When Sofie was seven years old her mainstream school decided that they could no longer cope with her in school. The annual review became an important conference. We had the bloke from special educational needs department there, her class teacher, all these other people and me sat there. It is unusual for me, in front of professionals but before the meeting ended I left in tears. They were quite concerned after that. It is a shame that you have to break down before they realise that this is a big issue.'

Mistrust between professions is unhelpful but 'replacing structural competition with cooperation requires collective action and collective action requires education and organisation' (Kohn 1986: 195). Rose analysed interviews from a range of professionals and states that:

> The themes of identity, expertise, territory and power that emerged from the analysis can be described as arising from the details of professional activity or role. What the professional does, who they interact with and how professional relationships are played out are all factors that have the potential to complicate processes of enacting collective preference. Issues around identity, expertise, territory and power that stem from these details mean that reaching a collective preference is not 'simply' a matter of establishing and committing to joint goals and plans.
>
> (Rose 2011: 160)

Attempts to encourage different public welfare agencies to work together includes provision for joint bids for project monies which occurred for the Children's Fund, Sure Start, and Educational Action Zones. Skrtic (1991) notes that sensitive management, clear organisation and well-defined goals can enable diverse groups of experts to work together successfully, as they did for the Apollo Space Project. For Skrtic 'collaboration and mutual adjustment' (1991: 171) can lead to the creation of new knowledge and skills as people are expected to 'adjust and revise their conventional theories and practices relative to those of their colleagues' and teams' progress on the tasks in hand' (1991: 171).

QUESTIONS

- With whom do you have an effective professional relationship? Outline how the relationship was developed.
- With which professionals might you build relationships and why?
- Give examples of multiagency projects taking place in your area of professional practice.

---

f) Building, using and maintaining professional networks

Sofie's mother built a supportive network across public welfare provision, voluntary organisations, and friends and family that enabled her to achieve fully signed educational provision for Sofie at a school within walking distance of home. Following a violent incident requiring police intervention, Sofie's mother was placed in accommodation near the deaf unit before moving again to a different county into local authority housing backing onto a fully signing school. The network of support surrounding Sofie and her mother has grown from her determination, her openness and her honesty.

Professionals also benefit from building supportive networks. Capra reinforces the value of networks noting 'the more complex its pattern of interconnections, the more resilient it will be' (1997: 295). Teachers may benefit from joining interschool networks or consortiums, attending courses, joining working groups, using websites or attending meetings to build, use and maintain networks. The school itself can be used as a venue for group activities, which can serve to broaden experiences for the school community.

QUESTIONS

- What are your current networks of personal and professional support?
- How might you develop one of these networks further, what other networks could you join?
- How might networks enhance your professional work?

CASE STUDY continued

The teachers at Sofie's mainstream school could no longer meet the needs of a child who was profoundly deaf. The trained expert teachers worked in one specialist unit for deaf children situated far away from the family home. At the review meeting the mother broke into tears, as she did not wish her child to board at school. She eventually gained the support of the council housing department and by engaging social services together with the police she was rehoused in a place from where her child could attend the deaf unit.

Conclusion

This chapter has outlined educational services for a child with profound hearing impairment illustrating challenges faced by the family in overseeing professional provision. The family encountered a range of educational professionals, health practitioners, voluntary workers, and officials working within social services.

Support for the family could have been more cohesive and effective if the professionals involved had developed effective strategies of communication. The following key areas are proposed as essential for the development of collaborative practice:

- active listening skills between client/professional and interprofessional colleagues;
- conversational competence;
- the capacity to use different modes of communication;

- a commitment to sharing knowledge with others involved;
- an ability to build effective professional relationships; and
- the capacity to build, use and maintain broad professional networks.

Professionals often use these skills as they work with clients. Interprofessional working requires these same skills to be taken into collaborative working relationships.

RECOMMENDED READING

- DfE (Department for Education) (2013) *Working Together to Safeguard Children* www.education.gov.uk. Accessed January 2014.
- Edwards A. (2009) *Improving Inter-Professional Collaborations: Multi-agency Working for Children's Wellbeing.* London: Routledge.
- Rose J. (2011) Dilemmas of inter-professional collaboration: can they be resolved? *Children and Society* **25**: 151–63.

References

Capra F. (1997) *The Web of Life: A New Synthesis of Mind and Matter.* London: Flamingo.

DCSF (Department for Children, Schools and Families) (2004) *Every Child Matters.* London: HMSO.

DfE (Department for Education) (2011) *Support and Aspiration: A New Approach to Special Educational Needs and Disability – A Consultation.* Norwich: The Stationery Office.

DfE (2012a) *Statutory Framework for the Early Years Foundation Stage; Setting the Standards for Learning, Development and Care for Children from Birth to Five.* Runcorn: DfE.

DfE (2012b) *Support and Aspiration: A New Approach to Special Educational Needs and Disability: Progress and Next Steps.* Runcorn: DfE.

DfE (2013a) *Working Together to Safeguard Children.* www.education.gov.uk. Accessed January 2013.

DfE (2013b) *Sure Start Children's Centres Statutory Guidance.* Runcorn: DfE.

DfE (2013c) *Children and Families Bill.* Norwich: The Stationery Office.

DfE/DH (Department for Education/Department of Health) (2013) *SEND Pathfinder Programme Report.* Runcorn: DfE.

DfEE (Department for Education and Employment) (2000a) *Educational Psychology Services (England): Current Role, Good Practice and Future Directions – The Research Report.* Nottingham: DfEE.

DfEE (2000b) *Sure Start: Making a Difference for Children and Families.* Nottingham: DfEE.

DfES (Department for Education and Skills) (2001) *Special Educational Needs Code of Practice.* London: HMSO.

Edwards A. (2009) *Improving Inter-Professional Collaborations: Multi-agency Working for Children's Wellbeing.* London: Routledge.

Farrell P., Woods K., Lewis S., Squires G., Rooney S. and O'Conner M. (2006) *A Review of the Functions and Contribution of Educational Psychologists in England and Wales in the Light of 'Every Child Matters: Change for Children'.* Nottingham: DfES.

Kohn A. (1986) *No Contest: The Case against Competition.* New York: Houghton Mifflin.

Roaf C. (2002) *Co-ordinating Services for Included Children: Joined Up Action.* Buckingham: Open University Press.

Rogers C. (1980) *A Way of Being.* Boston: Houghton Mifflin.

Rose J. (2011) Dilemmas of inter-professional collaboration: can they be resolved? *Children and Society* 25: 151–63.

Sellman D. (2010) Values and ethics in interprofessional working. In Pollard K.C., Thomas J. and Miers M. (eds) *Understanding Interprofessional Working in Health and Social Care: Theory and Practice.* Basingstoke: Palgrave Macmillan, pp. 156–70.

Skrtic T.M. (1991) The special education paradox: equity is the way to excellence. *Harvard Educational Review* 61: 148–206.

Svensson L.G. (1990) Knowledge as a professional resource: case studies of architects and psychologists at work. In Torstendahl R. and Burrage M. (eds) *The Formation of Professions.* London: Sage, pp. 51–70.

TA (Teaching Agency) (2011) www.education.gov.uk. Accessed November 2012.

Tarr J. (2003) *The Personal Qualities and Attributes of Professionals Working with Parents of Children with Special Educational Needs.* Unpublished doctoral thesis. Bristol: University of the West of England.

Vass G. (1991) Marginal dialogues, social positions and inequity in rhetorical resources. In Mettens R. and Vass G. (eds) *Sharing Mathematics Cultures.* Lewes: Falmer Press, pp. 214–31.

Young I.M. (2000) *Inclusion and Democracy.* Oxford: Oxford University Press.

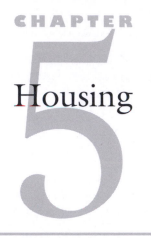

CHAPTER

Housing

Judith Ritchie and Ceri Victory

Introduction

The inter-relationship between health and housing has been recognised since Victorian times. During the 19th century improved sanitation and disposal of human waste, better housing construction and the reduction in overcrowding served to ameliorate housing conditions contributing to acute infectious diseases. Researchers in the late 20th and early 21st centuries have recognised continuing links between housing conditions and health (see, for example, Burridge and Ormandy 1993, Heywood and Turner 2007). Today it is chronic non-infectious conditions such as asthma that represent the primary cause of housing-related health problems, and the relationships between housing, health and socio-economic status are diverse and increasingly complex (Marmot 2010, Ormandy 2007).

The negative impacts of poor housing have been made clear in studies ranging over more than a decade (see, for example, Ineichen 1993, Ormandy 2007), which show that accommodation with cold, damp, mouldy conditions, overcrowding or poor repair has a detrimental effect on health. Housing stressors are shown to be associated with psychological distress and to contribute to mental health problems (Kearns and Smith 1993, Page 2002). In particular, there is evidence that poor or unsuitable housing has an adverse effect on the physical and mental health of children with disabilities and their families (Marsh, Gordon, Helsop and Pantazis 2000, Oldman and Beresford 2000).

It is clear from these studies that if people with health or social care needs are not housed appropriately there is a significant risk of deterioration in their health over a range of parameters. Correspondingly, research examining positive interventions (Beresford and Oldman 2002, Heywood and Turner 2007) has found that housing adaptations for people with disabilities successfully keep people out of hospital, reduce strain on carers, and promote social inclusion.

This chapter considers some of the difficulties people with health or social care needs might face in accessing accommodation appropriate to their needs. This encompasses people who are homeless or occupy poor quality accommodation, or those who require adaptations to the property or support or care in order for them to live independently.

Such individuals may be resident in the social, private rented or owner occupied sectors and it is important for professionals assisting in these cases to understand the nature of each sector. The majority of people in the United Kingdom (UK) still own their own home although the numbers continue to decline, going from 69.4 per cent in 2004 to 64.7 per cent in 2011(Wilcox and Pawson 2013). Eighteen per cent were renting from the social sector in 2011, a fairly steady figure since 2004, whereas in the same period the private rented sector has increased from 11.3 per cent to 17.4 per cent (Wilcox and Pawson 2013), and it is worth noting that, as the Localism Act 2011 (www.legislation. gov.uk) permits local authorities to discharge their duty to homeless applicants by housing them in the private sector, we may now see increasing numbers of vulnerable people, many with health or social care needs, housed in private rented accommodation.

Just as there is diversity of tenure, there is diversity within the housing profession, as described in this chapter and, consequently, a health or social care professional seeking to assist someone, will often need to work with a range of housing providers and other agencies to achieve their aims. The chapter starts by providing some detailed information about the organisations involved in both the provision and planning of housing and housing services in order to enhance the ability of other professionals to understand the operational boundaries and constraints within which housing professionals work.

Organisations involved in the provision and planning of housing and housing services

The provision of housing is overseen strategically by the relevant local authority. Local authorities are also providers of housing: general needs affordable (or social) housing is provided by local authorities or housing associations on a not-for-profit basis. Accommodation is allocated on the basis of housing need and providers are charged with supporting people in maintaining their tenancies. Housing associations are also significant providers of supported housing alongside charities and other voluntary organisations, and the private sector is playing an increasing role in the provision of care homes, other specialist supported accommodation as well as increased provision of rented general needs accommodation. Private landlords generally operate for profit and are less regulated than social landlords.

Local authorities

The importance of council housing in numerical terms has diminished since the 1980s. All local housing authorities, however, retain a strategic role in relation to housing in the local area. As part of this role the authority must produce a number of strategies in collaboration with other statutory and voluntary agencies. These strategies are outlined below:

a) *Sustainable Communities Strategy* requires local authorities 'to set the overall strategic direction and long-term vision for the economic, social and environmental well- being of a local area' (DCLG 2008: 26).
b) *Housing strategy* which covers all aspects of housing in its area including an analysis of all housing markets and an assessment of the housing needs of all sections of the community. The Housing Strategy gives details of local housing priorities, setting out current and anticipated housing needs and indicating where resources are to be targeted.
c) *Homelessness strategy:* Brought in by the Homelessness Act 2002 (www.legislation.gov.uk), this document sets out plans for combating and preventing homelessness. It identifies likely homelessness levels in the future and resources available to prevent homelessness and secure suitable accommodation. Local authorities have a duty to administer homelessness legislation, and must offer advice to anyone who is homeless or threatened with homelessness. Housing, health and social care professionals can effectively work together to ensure not only that appropriate decisions are made with homeless individuals, but also that resources are used effectively and efficiently.
d) *Supporting people strategy:* The Supporting People programme began in 2003 in order to coordinate funding and provision of housing-related support services (defined and clearly distinguished from the provision of personal care). Its principal aim was 'to help vulnerable people avoid or delay entry into institutional services, and to live as independently as possible for as long as possible' (Sitra 2011: 2).

Registered providers

The term *registered provider* (previously registered social landlord) is used to describe organisations providing affordable (or social) housing. Such organisations operate within the voluntary sector, and many are registered charities. The registered providers that health and social care professionals will most commonly encounter are housing associations. Some offer general needs housing whereas others specialise in housing for a particular client group and may provide services *not* tied to accommodation such as floating or visiting support.

Private sector landlords

The use of private rented sector housing often forms part of a local authority's homelessness strategy. Reliance on this sector is likely to increase since the Localism Act 2011. However, finding private sector rented accommodation to meet the health needs of individuals is difficult and the potential for making adaptations will depend on the willingness of the landlord to permit such work. Research by Carlton, Heywood, Izuhara *et al.* (2003) into the living conditions of older people in the private rented sector identified problems that give serious cause for concern for the health and well-being of some vulnerable people who live in this sector. Much of the private sector is unregulated, despite growing calls for this to change in order to offer protection to those vulnerable people housed, sometimes unsatisfactorily, in private rented properties (Crisis 2010, DCLG 2009).

Voluntary organisations

Voluntary, not-for-profit organisations are significant providers both of accommodation with support and of floating support or care services. Organisations may focus on one client group, for example, the single homeless, young people or those with mental health problems.

Interagency working

We have observed above that in many situations housing, health and social care professionals may need to work together in order to address housing needs adequately and appropriately. Means, Brenton, Harrison and Heywood (1997) note that this type of interagency working may be required in gaining access to social housing, staying put and providing care and support packages.

Gaining access to social housing

In many cases it may be appropriate for people with health or social care needs, whose housing needs are not being met in the private sector, to access general needs accommodation in the social sector. A care or support package may then be put in place to support those individuals to remain in their home (see below). Access to general needs social housing usually requires an assessment of the applicant's housing need, taking into account such factors as the condition of their current accommodation, their age and mental and physical health, and whether they are pregnant or have dependent children. Where applications are made on health grounds, a reference may be required from a health professional stating that the current housing is having a detrimental effect on the health of the applicant (or a household member) or that change of housing is required in order to meet the applicant's health needs. Once assessed and found eligible, applicants are placed on a waiting list or housing register in order of priority. In some areas there is a separate list for each housing organisation, with varying eligibility criteria; other areas operate a Common Housing Register where one application only is required to be housed by any local social housing provider. It is important to note that the Localism Act 2011 has given local authorities greater freedom to set their own housing allocation policies, although they must still give reasonable preference to those in housing need. The published tenancy strategy will be a key document for those supporting someone seeking social rented accommodation.

Choice based lettings

There is a belief that allocation according to housing need has led to a concentration of deprived households on unpopular estates, thus contributing to social exclusion and neighbourhood decline (Brown, Hunt and Yates 2000). In response recent governments have promoted a policy of choice, a radical change in the way social housing is allocated. Many local authorities and housing associations now operate Choice Based Lettings Systems (ODPM 2004) where housing applicants are assessed and placed within a category: urgent housing need, a housing need; and no immediate housing need. Available properties are then advertised with information about who would be eligible to apply. The major change is that applicants need actively to apply for a property, rather than wait to be allocated accommodation.

This may present a significant barrier for those who experience difficulties of any sort in understanding or engaging with such systems. Concern has been expressed (CSIP/NIMHE 2006, Grannum 2005) that the vulnerable could be disadvantaged by such systems, and interagency collaboration is likely to be required to ensure that people's needs do not go unnoticed. In particular, applicants may need active, practical support to engage proactively and effectively with the allocation system. It is therefore important that professionals are familiar with their local allocation systems and with the provision made for vulnerable applicants to engage with these systems. The significance of informed support for vulnerable applicants is evident when the scale of the challenge involved in securing social housing is realised: in Bristol in March 2012, for example, there were 16,231 households on the housing register, set against an annual vacancy rate of 2,500–3,000 properties (HomeChoice 2012).

Homeless applicants

Particular provisions are made for applicants who are deemed homeless. Local authorities have a statutory duty to advise and assist all homeless people but only those who are judged to be eligible (which depends on citizenship/immigration status), unintentionally homeless and in priority need will be offered housing. Others are simply entitled to information and assistance. The Housing Act 1996 and the Homelessness Act 2002 contain definitions of what it means to be *unintentionally homeless* and *in priority need* and it should be noted that those who are literally roofless make up only a small percentage of the homeless (Audit Commission 2003). Health and social care workers may have contact with many people who are homeless, because they live in unsuitable housing. They may be in danger from violence or threats of violence, staying with friends temporarily, or being threatened with eviction, and each of these situations renders a person homeless. However, while a local authority *may* rehouse those who are homeless but not in priority need, if there is housing available, there is no statutory *duty* for them to do so.

Access to supported housing

In some cases specialist housing offering integrated care or support services may be needed. The way in which specialist housing can be accessed varies depending on location; consequently, it is again important that professionals who come into contact with those in housing need familiarise themselves with local application or referral processes. Commonly, services will accept referrals only (rather than direct applications), so having clear protocols and building relationships with the people who work in specific individual services may be important. In some instances referrals may be made direct to services but in others centralised systems, or gateways, have been set up. Centralised referral systems offer professionals the benefit of a single source of information about services and enable multiple applications with a single referral, but they do potentially reduce the ability to influence outcomes by building relationships with individual services.

CASE STUDY: Joe Green

Joe Green, a white male now in his mid-20s, left home at 17 because of an abusive stepfather. He lived with friends until he found work and could afford to rent a private sector bedsit. Things began to go wrong when he met an older group of young men and was drawn into their heavy drinking lifestyle. For Joe, perhaps because of unresolved issues in his past, this quickly became an alcohol dependency. As a result he lost his job, was evicted from his bedsit, and because as a private sector tenant there was no automatic recourse to housing advice, Joe thought that, as a young single person, there was no one to offer him help.

Joe began living on the street. He heard about a *one-stop-shop* run by the local council giving advice to homeless people. The one-stop-shop is an interagency project with representatives from the local authority's homelessness team, social services and the health service working together in the same building in order to provide a single point of assessment for an individual. Unfortunately, Joe, who did not cope well with being *street homeless*, only went to the advice centre when drunk and became abusive when waiting to be seen. Consequently he was repeatedly turned away.

An individual's needs are often complex, and despite the provision of services such as this multiagency advice centre it may be problematic to connect the individual with the service.

QUESTIONS

- What do you consider to be Joe's needs at this time?
- What service providers would need to be involved in meeting his needs?
- How might Joe best access these services?

CASE STUDY continued

Joe is met by a street outreach worker employed by a voluntary agency acting as part of the council's strategy for combating street homelessness. The outreach worker makes an appointment for Joe to attend a meeting at a day centre for homeless people where his needs can be assessed. Joe misses several appointments, but does eventually attend and has his housing, health and support needs assessed. A member of the team also gives him a formal alcohol assessment.

Having made contact with the day centre, Joe begins to use it and accesses the services of the nurses who attend the centre on a twice-weekly basis. A four-way meeting is organised between Joe, the hostel nurse, the outreach worker and the alcohol worker. It is agreed that Joe is ready for a detoxification programme, and a place is found for him in a residential centre with a subsequent referral to a long stay hostel where he would be able to stay for up to two years.

It is important that Joe receives treatment quickly, and this is dependent on the availability of places in a detoxification unit. Following detoxification, Joe will need to be placed in a hostel, and it is at this point that interagency working often breaks down. Hostels are usually run by Housing Associations or voluntary organisations, and each tends to have its own referral criteria. One problem for health and social care workers is knowing which hostels are available and the details of their particular referral criteria. As part of their strategic housing duty, local authorities should make such information available, and will maintain a website providing information about local provision providing support for vulnerable people. If such information is lacking it is the strategic housing team of the local authority who should be contacted.

CASE STUDY continued

Being placed in the hostel is very much a starting point for Joe. His needs are assessed by his key worker in the hostel, and a package of support is agreed.

He will be registered with a GP and could be referred to a community mental health team.

Once Joe is ready to move on from the hostel, he will be reassessed, and should be referred to some form of floating support to help maintain his tenancy.

Too often, placing an individual in a hostel is seen as a success, and the momentum is lost in tackling issues that need to be addressed. Effective interagency working can make the difference between the hostel placement being a temporary shelter and being a time of transformation. Hostel workers alone are unlikely to have the skills to meet all of Joe's needs. For example, Joe still has issues related to his abusive stepfather and access to floating support is essential in helping him towards independent living.

Staying put

Another important interface between housing and health and social care occurs when people find that their home itself has become disabling. This can happen at any time through illness or accident, but is more likely as people grow older. Social services and the occupational therapy service are often the first point of contact, but housing has an important role to play.

For someone living in social housing, it is possible that the landlord has a budget for minor aids and adaptations and may assist with necessary alterations. Disabled Facilities Grants may also be available for alterations or adaptations. Alternatively transfer into a more suitable home may be possible and the formal input of a health or social care professional is likely to be essential to expedite this.

People who own their own homes or live in the private rented sector can access assistance through a home improvement agency (HIA). HIAs do not fund works but enable people to obtain funding through grants, loans or equity release. They also help plan required works and negotiate with builders, working with individuals to maintain their homes to a decent standard. HIAs were incorporated into the Supporting People programme and so, like other housing-related support services, are now vulnerable to funding reductions following the removal of the Supporting People ring-fenced funds.

Care and support packages

There are many instances when people living in their own home require care or support in order to remain there; equally it may be determined through assessment that their needs can be better met in specialised accommodation such as supported housing or a care home. The significance of taking a joined-up approach to meeting housing, care and support needs has been recognised by initiatives such as the Health and Social Care Change Agent Team (CAT), which aims to reduce the number of delayed hospital discharges and associated arrangements. Hospital discharge planning is a priority for all services because of the serious consequences of delayed or inappropriate discharge on both service user and provider, as reflected in the fact that the Delayed Discharges Act 2003 (www.legislation.gov.uk) means that NHS costs for delayed discharge must be reimbursed by social services departments, if such delays are due to their inaction. Acknowledging the important role of housing in this process, CAT set up a Housing Learning and Improvement Network in November 2002 and continues to provide a useful source of information of best practice in this area of work via the Department of Health website (www.dh.gov.uk).

Personalisation

The personalisation agenda (DH 2006, 2007) places an even greater emphasis on the need for all services to work together in order to achieve person-centred service delivery.

For housing providers personalisation includes:

■ tailoring support to people's individual needs to enable them to live full, independent lives
■ choice in how and where they could live and to ensure that homes are well designed, flexible and accessible
■ developing ways to respond to personalisation through specialist housing
■ ensuring that people have access to information and advice to make good decisions about their care and support
■ finding new collaborative ways of working that support people to actively engage in the design, delivery and evaluation of services (SCIE 2009).

Tailored support and care

Provision for older people is an area where tailored support and care packages have become particularly significant during recent years. Sheltered housing, or independent accommodation with warden support, became less popular for this age group from the 1980s as a result of increased longevity and better health in old age. The move into sheltered accommodation often now comes at a time of crisis when people are far frailer than previously with the result that a rather different form of service is required. Sheltered housing now comes with varying levels of support, and some schemes have been created specifically to meet the needs of the frail older person. The role of the warden in such schemes is as coordinator of complex interagency services delivering personalised combinations of support and care. Effective interagency working in this context enables people to maintain a degree of independence and stay out of residential care for longer than would otherwise be the case. There are many other contexts – for example, services for people with learning disabilities or mental health issues – where similar results can be achieved.

CASE STUDY: Rose Perkins

Rose Perkins, a 72-year-old widow who is blind but otherwise in good health, was recently admitted to hospital for a medical condition. She had been living in the home of relatives for the past 10 years although she had experienced some conflict with them. She is ready for discharge, but her family has refused to take her back as they plan to move to a smaller house and will no longer be able to care for her.

Rose is accustomed to undertaking personal and domestic tasks. Until her admission she was able to bathe without attendance, did the washing up and cooked using gas. The shopping, cleaning and other domestic activities were done by her relatives.

As you work with Rose you will need to identify her needs and her wishes but it is important that you are informed about possible options.

QUESTIONS

- What sort of accommodation do you think might be suitable to meet Rose's needs on discharge from hospital?
- Whom would you contact to try to assist Rose in identifying such accommodation?
- What assistance might Rose require from health and social care professionals to find appropriate accommodation?
- What level of support might you need to think about with Rose if she wished to live independently?

CASE STUDY continued

Following an application made on her behalf by her relatives and a community care assessment by a social worker, Rose was assessed as an urgent medical priority case. She moved into a first floor self-contained one bedroom housing association flat in extra care sheltered accommodation within one month of applying to the local authority.

Rose is delighted with her current accommodation, enjoys its spaciousness and comfort and finds the carers attached to the scheme 'wonderful – not too interfering but always there when needed'. She has not cooked for herself since she moved because there is no gas supply and she is frightened of electric cookers. She has meals delivered to her flat each day, and a friend of the family helps her with washing, cleaning, shopping and collecting her pension.

Rose still lives within walking distance of where she has lived for the past 50 years and has maintained her local contacts, as well as befriending other residents and attending a range of activities organised in the sheltered scheme.

She believes that her health and overall quality of life have improved as she no longer has to deal with difficult personality differences on a daily basis and revels in being able to live independently. Her use of health services comprises regular visits to the practice nurse for blood pressure checks and she has significantly reduced her number of GP appointments since the move. However, her use of other services has increased, as she has twice-daily visits from scheme care assistants and meals delivered. She arranges and pays for her home help service privately.

Whether or not Rose will be able to remain in her flat will depend on her ongoing capacity to care for herself and the level of frailty the scheme is able to cope with. Interagency working is vital in sheltered accommodation to ensure that an individual's capacity to cope is carefully monitored so that they can be moved to a higher care environment when necessary.

Conclusion

Partnership between housing, health and social care agencies has been fraught with difficulties in the past, and effective interagency working continues to be difficult to achieve. Arblaster, Conway, Foreman and Hawtin highlighted the contradictory nature of government policies such as the competition in public services, customer choice and reducing public expenditure that impact on 'effective collaboration between housing, health and social care' (1996: xiv). Their work emphasised the need for sufficient time and resources to be devoted to working in partnership, for better communication between agencies and service users, and for joint interagency procedures to be developed. Writing in 2011 at a time when there were further calls for cuts in government expenditure, Glasby, Dickinson and Miller stated, 'Above all, they will need to realise that health and social care *have* to work together to support people with complex needs, and that cuts in spending make joint working even harder but even more important' (2011: 7).

One of the most problematic areas for partnership working, and an area where effective partnership is essential, is in meeting the complex needs of some homeless people. Effective interagency working becomes especially difficult to achieve when the organisations involved work within geographical boundaries that are not co-terminus, and when the organisations have different objectives and ways of working with the same client group. Both Joe Green and Rose Perkins were appropriately rehoused and received the support they required. This is not always the case and many people fall through the support networks, often with dire consequences. There are a number of publications about interagency working that should be helpful for practitioners in this field, in particular those by Means *et al.* (1997), Arblaster Conway Foreman and Hawtin (1998), Balloch and Taylor (2001) and Cameron, McDonald, Turner and Lloyd (2007). Although effective partnership working is difficult to achieve it is nevertheless possible given sufficient commitment and resources.

RECOMMENDED READING

- Glasby J., Dickinson H. and Miller R. (2011) Partnership working in England: Where we are now and where we have come from? *International Journal of Integrated Care* **11** (Special 10th Anniversary Edition): e002. www.ijic.org. Accessed February 2013.
- Housing Learning and Improvement Network policy briefing (April 2009) *Living Well with Dementia: A National Dementia Strategy*. www.housinglin.org.uk. Accessed February 2013.
- SCIE (Social Care Institute for Excellence) (2009) *At a Glance 8: Personalisation Briefing: Implications for Housing Providers*. London: SCIE.

References

Arblaster L., Conway J., Foreman A. and Hawtin M. (1996) *Asking the Impossible? Interagency Working to Address the Housing, Health and Social Care Needs of People in Ordinary Housing*. Bristol: Policy Press.

Arblaster L., Conway J., Foreman A. and Hawtin M. (1998) *Achieving the Impossible: Interagency Collaboration to Address the Housing, Health and Social Care Needs of People Able to Live in Ordinary Housing*. Bristol: Policy Press.

Audit Commission (2003) *Homelessness: Responding to the New Agenda*. London: Audit Commission.

Balloch S. and Taylor M. (eds) (2001) *Partnership Working: Policy and Practice*. Bristol: Policy Press.

Beresford B. and Oldman C. (2002) *Housing Matters: National Evidence Related to Disabled Children and their Housing*. Bristol: Policy Press.

Brown T., Hunt R. and Yates N. (2000) *Lettings: A Question of Choice*. Coventry: Chartered Institute of Housing.

Burridge R. and Ormandy D. (eds) (1993) *Unhealthy Housing: Research, Remedies, Reform*. London: E and F N Spon.

Cameron A., McDonald G., Turner W. and Lloyd L. (2007) The challenges of joint working: lessons from the Supporting People Health Pilot Evaluation. *International Journal of Integrated Care* 7 October–December: e39. www.ijic.org. Accessed February 2013.

Carlton N., Heywood F., Izuhara M., Pannell J., Fear T. and Means R. (2003) *The Harassment and Abuse of Older People in the Private Rented Sector*. Bristol: Policy Press.

Crisis (2010) *Crisis Policy Briefing: Housing and the Private Rented Sector*. London: Crisis.

CSIP/NIMHE (Care Services Improvement Partnership/National Institute for Mental Health in England) (2006) *Choice Based Lettings for People with Mental Health Problems*. National Mental Health Development Unit. www.housinglin.org.uk. Accessed June 2013.

DCLG (Department for Communities and Local Government) (2008) *The Strategic Housing Role of Local Authorities: Power and Duties*. London: HMSO.

DCLG (2009) *The Private Rented Sector: Professionalism and Quality. Government Response to the Rugg Review*. London: HMSO.

DH (Department of Health) (2006) *Our Health, Our Care, Our Say: A New Direction of Community Services*. London: The Stationery Office.

DH (2007) *Putting People First: A Shared Vision and Commitment to the Transformation of Adult Social Care*. London: The Stationery Office.

Glasby J., Dickinson H. and Miller R. (2011) Partnership working in England: where we are now and where we have come from. *International Journal of Integrated Care* 11 (Special 10th Anniversary Edition) e002. www.ijic.org. Accessed February 2013.

Grannum C. (2005) *A Question of Choice*. London: Shelter.

Heywood F. and Turner L. (2007) *Better Outcomes Lower Costs. Implications for Health and Social Care Budgets of Investment in Housing Adaptations, Improvements and Equipment: A Review of the Evidence*. Bristol: School for Policy Studies.

HomeChoice (2012) Available at www.homechoicebristol.co.uk/.

Ineichen B. (1993) *Homes and Health: How Housing and Health Interact*. London: E. and F.N. Spon.

Kearns R.A. and Smith C.J. (1993) Housing stressors and mental health among marginalised urban populations. *Area* **25**(3): 267–68.

Marmot M. (2010) *Fair Society, Healthy Lives: The Marmot Review*. London: University College London.

Marsh A., Gordon D., Helsop P. and Pantazis C. (2000) Housing deprivation and health: a longitudinal analysis. *Housing Studies* **15**: 411–28.

Means R., Brenton M., Harrison L. and Heywood F. (1997) *Making Partnerships Work in Community Care: A Guide for Practitioners in Housing, Health and Social Services*. Bristol: Policy Press.

ODPM (Office of the Deputy Prime Minister) (2004) *Piloting Choice-Based Lettings: An Evaluation*. Housing Research Summary No. 208. London: ODPM.

Oldman C. and Beresford B. (2000) Home, sick home: using the housing experiences of disabled children to suggest a new theoretical framework. *Housing Studies* **15**: 429–42.

Ormandy D. (2007) *Housing Conditions and Health*. In Dowler E. and Spencer N.J. (eds) *Changing Health Inequalities: From Acheson to 'Choosing Health'*. Bristol: Policy Press, pp. 111–27.

Page A. (2002) Poor housing and mental health in the UK: changing the focus for intervention. *International Journal of Environmental Health Research* 1(1). www.cieh.org. Accessed February 2013.

SCIE (Social Care Institute for Excellence) (2009) *At a Glance 8: Personalisation Briefing: Implications for Housing Providers.* London: SCIE.

Sitra (2011) *Valuing Supporting People: Use of the Capgemini Tool in Housing Support Services.* London: Sitra.

Wilcox S. and Pawson H. (eds) (2013) *UK Housing Review* 2010/11. Chartered Institute of Housing.

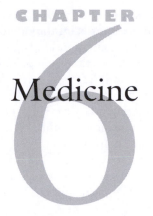

Medicine

Lindsey Dow and Nansi Evans

Introduction

Medical practitioners see patients with mental and physical health issues from across the age range in both community and hospital settings. Medicine is one of the oldest professions in the world yet it rarely stands still. It continues to develop within discrete specialities, each recognising the value and importance of working collaboratively with other professional groups to provide treatment and care. Rather than attempting to capture the full extent of medical practice, this chapter offers a brief overview of medicine, focusing on the roles and responsibilities of medical practitioners, before introducing two case studies drawn from general practice to illustrate the contribution of doctors to inter-professional working. Despite being a specific example of medical practice, general practice provides an overview of much that is common in medicine, particularly in relation to the attributes required for sucessful interprofessional working. It should be noted that while there is some debate about the most appropriate term for those who seek care from doctors, in this chapter we use the term 'patient' throughout.

The role of medical practitioners

Most people are familiar with doctors diagnosing and treating those who experience ill health, as they will usually have encountered them in primary care settings, that is, at general practitioner (GP) surgeries or out-of-hours centres, or in hospital (secondary care). Primary care accounts for 90 per cent of patient consultations (The King's Fund 2011). When someone consults a GP about a symptom, for example joint pain, the doctor tries to identify possible causes through listening to the patient, asking questions and undertaking an examination. Overall, the aim is to relieve the pain, but usually pain signifies a problem. The outcome may be referral to secondary care for investigations and/or prescription of a drug or a non-drug treatment such as physiotherapy. Doctors in both primary and secondary care may discuss other options such as lifestyle change, for example, losing weight. Hence a consultation includes obtaining information about the problem, communication about the diagnosis and treatment options, and negotiation regarding the most appropriate option, sometimes supplemented with written information. Doctors work in partnership with patients, and support them to maintain their health.

Education

Most medical students study for five years before qualifying. A strategy to widen access has meant some graduate entrants enrol on a four-year accelerated programme, while individuals without A-levels may enter an extended course. Many students incorporate an intercalated year for another degree in a related subject of interest, for example, neuroscience or medical ethics, midway through the course. Medical schools' curricula differ in the amount of clinical contact in the first two years and whether or not the course is problem-based (Azer 2008). The Medical Schools Council is currently (2013) exploring common assessment materials for UK medical schools.

All doctors continue to study after qualifying in order to maintain standards. Following undergraduate education, doctors spend two years in the Foundation Training Programme, registering with the General Medical Council (GMC) after the first year. A few move into non-clinical roles, but most then train for general or hospital practice. GP training programmes usually take three years, including time in approved hospital posts. Training in a hospital speciality like paediatrics requires core and speciality training over approximately eight years. This time allows for development of specialist skills and opportunities to undertake research and/or obtain further academic qualifications. During training, medical students and doctors are encouraged to develop additional skills in teaching, management and leadership (GMC 2012). Junior doctors are trained under close supervision so that they fufil competencies and demonstrate appropriate professional behaviour (GMC 2006).

A survey conducted by the Postgraduate Medical Education and Training Board (PMETB 2009) (now merged with the GMC) showed that trainees had few opportunities for multi- or interprofessional learning. A subsequent evaluation of the Foundation Programme (Collins 2010) and a report into the state of medical education and practice (GMC 2011) both recommended educational opportunities for foundation doctors to develop the skills needed to work in multidisciplinary teams and environments.

The GMC requires all practising doctors to hold a licence and to undergo annual appraisals leading to revalidation every five years. Doctors are appraised by a colleague trained in the process, using a structured approach to produce a development plan for the year ahead. Revalidation includes evidence of maintenance/acquisition of knowledge and skills, and positive/negative feedback from colleagues and patients.

More women than men have entered medical school since the 1990s and comprise more than 40 per cent of practising doctors in England (Elston 2009). General practice has had a more flexible approach to work-life balance than hospital specialities and thus has attracted more women doctors. However, secondary care has responded by developing flexible training, and part-time doctors in training are common in hospitals. In secondary care, women have tended to choose specialities with relatively predictable working patterns, but some now enter 'tougher' specialities such as orthopaedics and cardiac surgery. The traditional model of doctors is changing and some doctors even combine medicine with a non-medical career such as art or journalism.

Working patterns

In 2009, the European Working Time Directive came into force, reducing junior doctors' maximum number of working hours to 48 hours per week. This highlighted difficulties of adequate time for training, and remains a major challenge for the profession and for the National Health Service (NHS). Shift work has meant that junior doctors spend less time in permanent teams during their first two years, the intensity of work has increased and it can be more difficult to build working relationships with colleagues. The European Working Time Directive has contributed to the development of enhanced roles for other health professionals, who sometimes acquire an advanced skill traditionally the preserve of doctors, for example, physiotherapists giving joint injections. This has led to some doctors feeling they lack sufficient experience or opportunities to practise during training because procedures are often performed by other professionals (PMETB 2009).

GPs were traditionally self-employed and contracted to provide NHS services but more than 20 per cent are now salaried and employed by a practice or primary care organisation (NHS 2010). Others work as sessional GPs, perhaps for an out-of-hours service. GPs may work from premises with a primary care team which includes both clinical and administrative staff. GPs can opt out of certain services such as antenatal care and may choose to provide enhanced services such as specialised care of the homeless. In addition, GPs are encouraged to attain certain standards based on best available evidence, for example, in clinical areas such as diabetes and coronary heart disease.

The Health and Social Care Act 2012 (www.legislation.gov.uk) outlines a series of NHS reforms, including the creation of GP-led clinical commissioning groups to work with managers and hospital doctors to commission services for patients. This involves doctors taking on more of a management role. Traditionally there have been conflicting priorities between doctors and NHS managers about how limited funds should be spent. The underlying principles of increased clinical leadership and public involvement are sound, but there is ongoing debate about how these structures will work in practice, as well as concerns about perceived trends towards destabilising the NHS and privatising health care services (McLellan, Middleton and Godlee 2012). Doctors must declare a conflict of interest should they be involved in both commissioning and providing a service.

The responsibilities of medical practitioners

Doctors manage the medical treatment of patients who may be acutely ill and expected to recover, who are terminally ill, or who experience chronic disease. Increasingly in primary care, doctors work to prevent disease, for example, treating high blood pressure to reduce the risk of stroke. The GMC (2006) sets out their duties and responsibilities. Essential elements include professional competence, good relationships with patients and colleagues, and observance of professional and ethical obligations.

GPs are often the first point of contact for people of all ages with a wide range of needs resulting from any combination of physical, psychological, social and emotional problems. GPs share the workload with colleagues. In primary care, practice nurses lead clinics managing a range of chronic diseases, such as asthma and diabetes, and are involved in minor injury services. Nurse practitioners have more responsibility, particularly in primary care, for example, walk-in centres, but also as hospital specialist nurses. The latter can diagnose and treat within their expertise, working closely with their medical colleagues, for example, running out-patient clinics for patients with a particular condition, such as rheumatology.

Doctors also refer patients to other professionals, such as physiotherapists or social workers. The referring doctor retains overall medical responsibility for the patient and must be satisfied that other professionals are appropriately qualified and professionally accountable (GMC 2006).

Interprofessional working

Interprofessional working is increasingly common as a means of delivering health care (Watts 2012). With an ageing population, more patients have complex needs that require an integrated response from a range of different professions. Good team work has been linked to better outcomes for patients, both clinical and in terms of patient satisfaction (Grumbach and Bodenheimer 2004). Each professional brings different expertise; therefore an interprofessional team can usually provide a more appropriate response than doctors working alone. In some hospital practice areas, for example rehabilitation, doctors may work more closely with other professionals within the team than with other doctors outside their speciality. Doctors remain accountable for providing medical care within the team and for their own professional conduct.

Successful interprofessional working requires effective communication and a willingness to listen to others and modify opinions (Vyt 2008). Working with different professionals can be challenging if there has been little opportunity for collaboration during undergraduate education. The GMC (2009) has identified a range of relevant outcomes for medical graduates with respect to interprofessional working. These include:

- understanding and respecting other professionals' roles and expertise;
- understanding how effective interdisciplinary team work contributes to the delivery of safe and high quality care;
- passing on information and handing over care appropriately, so as to optimise patients' interests;

■ demonstrating the ability to build team capacity and positive working relationships with medical and non-medical colleagues.

There continues to be discussion about whether patient-held records facilitate communication between professionals and help involve patients in their own care (Ko, Turner, Jones and Hill 2010). This already happens in maternity care, where community midwives, GPs and hospital staff use the same set of paper records which the pregnant woman carries; and in the intermediate care team setting, where patients with acute illnesses receive specialised care at home from a team who all use the same set of records kept with patients.

Most GP records are computerised. Computerised records have the potential to improve interprofessional working and to allow better information flow between primary and secondary care (Ward and Innes 2003). With modern technology, even with staff working from different bases, it is important that there is one site for storing related information about an individual patient so that everyone can access it and make informed decisions. However, this needs to be balanced with the need for confidentiality as not all information is relevant to every professional involved with patient care.

Twenty-first century patients have excellent access to information and increasingly high expectations of their doctors. Nevertheless, patients continue to trust their doctors (Ipsos MORI 2011) and many expect consultations to be confidential; they occasionally ask that certain sensitive details are not recorded or shared with other professionals (for example, information regarding a sexually transmitted disease). Should other professionals be involved in care, the doctor will explain to the patient the benefit of sharing relevant information but cannot normally disclose such information without the patient's consent. This can cause conflict as care of the patient is the doctor's first concern while also being required to work with colleagues to best serve the patient's interest (GMC 2006). However, in exceptional circumstances, the benefit of disclosure for the public may outweigh the patient's interests (for example, if a patient has a communicable disease). If a doctor feels there is a conflict of interest, is unable to persuade the patient to allow information to be shared, and is in doubt as to how to proceed, it is advisable to seek advice from one of the professional bodies, such as the Medical Protection Society, which specialise in issues of law and ethics relating to medical practice (MPS 2012).

The sharing of responsibility is a key element of interprofessional working (Vyt 2008). The primary aim of interprofessional working is a better outcome for patients but there are also benefits of improved support and shared decision-making for professionals involved in the often difficult and demanding work of health and social care. Each profession has a particular approach and while some overlap exists in, for example, assessment processes, there may sometimes be clashes of treatment priorities for an individual patient. For instance, doctors may wish to treat a patient with lung cancer in whom the chance of success is low and where the treatment has significant side effects. The patient may wish to leave the decision for treatment with the doctor. The nurses who care for the patient on a daily basis may feel the level of suffering from side effects is so great that treatment should not continue. These differences of perspective are important; nurses often hold patient comfort, dignity, lack of pain and suffering as priority values. These values are also a priority for doctors but are judged, in this case, against evidence of the cancer responding to intensive treatment. Doctors are trained to deal with risk and uncertainty in clinical situations, and may be more comfortable than other health care professions in deviating from guidelines if the clinical situation demands it. Successful interprofessional working relies upon sharing patient concerns as well as professional perspectives, values and beliefs (Molyneux 2001, Vyt 2008).

There can also be challenges when roles and status change. For example, many doctors have been concerned at the extended role of nurses who prescribe medication after shorter training in therapeutics than doctors undertake. Prescribing has become more complex, with many patients on multiple medications, and increased potential for serious interactions which even the most experienced prescriber will sometimes fail to anticipate. However, as professionals, nurses are accountable for their prescribing actions and are responsible for acting within their area of expertise and training.

Some doctors also work with charities representing patients and their carers to define standards of care and give information and support. Organisations such as the Stroke Association, Age UK and Macmillan Cancer Support provide training for specialists, fund research and work with different professionals to improve patient care.

CASE STUDY: Christine Braithwaite

Christine Braithwaite is a 45-year-old woman of African Caribbean origin with metastatic breast cancer diagnosed five years ago. She is a single mother with two sons, aged 12 and 15. A week ago she learned the disease has progressed, further chemotherapy will not be of benefit and she may have only weeks left to live. She has been able to manage so far with the support of a Macmillan nurse, GP contact and regular oncology specialist care. This morning her Macmillan nurse asks the GP to visit because Christine is reporting increased back pain. The GP finds Christine up and about but in pain. This is their first meeting since her recent prognosis. Examination reveals that the pain is from known secondary bone cancer and the doctor advises adjusting medication. Christine wants to talk about what is likely to happen. Her concern is who will look after her and how her children will cope. Their father lives away but sees the boys regularly; she has a small network of friends who help with the children. Her youngest son is not settling well at high school and does not get on with Christine's partner, who lives locally, but has his own problems. Christine gets upset thinking about the future and ends the conversation. She wants to carry on as normal for as long as possible, and doesn't want too many reminders of her illness.

QUESTION

■ Which other professionals could help Christine?

■ Most GP practices have a register of palliative patients and hold regular multidisciplinary team meetings. The GP should alert the out-of-hours service of all palliative patients to ensure prompt and appropriate care.

■ Christine's Macmillan nurse provides clinical advice, emotional, practical and financial support and advice, and may be the best person to keep contact wih her until she wants to engage with other members of the team.

■ District nurses can assess nursing needs and apply for funding for continuing health care should Christine decide she wishes to spend her last days at home.

■ Social workers may need to be involved in any child care issues, or if non-nursing care is needed.

■ Physiotherapists and occupational therapists may help maintain Christine at home.

■ The pharmacist may need to know that she is a palliative patient.

■ The consultant oncologist is available to respond to any questions the GP or Macmillan nurse have.

■ The Department of Health has published an *End of Life Care Strategy* to support health and social care teams in England and Wales (DH 2008). Similar strategies, involving a multidisciplinary approach, are in place in Scotland (NHS Scotland 2008) and Northern Ireland (DHSSPS 2010).

CASE STUDY continued

Christine has a few good weeks and spends time with family and friends. She keeps in touch by phone with her Macmillan nurse and eventually feels able to talk with her GP and Macmillan nurse about her wish to die at home. The GP suggests that a 'Just in Case' box of drugs, including morphine for pain control, be left in the home should Christine suddenly deteriorate out-of-hours, and liaises with the local pharmacist who provides this service. The Macmillan nurse also advises a community DNAR (do not attempt resuscitation) form be kept at home so that, should an ambulance be called in an emergency, the crew will not start cardio-pulmonary resuscitation inappropriately. The Macmillan nurse facilitates Christine's talk to the boys' father, and her concerns for their future. The Macmillan nurse spends time with the younger son, and with Christine's permission, liaises with the school nurse to support him.

One day, Christine suddenly becomes extremely short of breath. A different GP visits her. Christine does not want to go to hospital, but the GP advises that an X-ray might help determine the problem. She has fluid around the lung, which is drained. She spends two days in hospital and her sister comes to stay. Christine now needs intermittent oxygen and stronger pain medication. Her main worry is her children, but she knows her disease is progressing and her time with them is short. She does not know whether it is better to transfer to a hospice, about 20 miles from her home, or to go home (which she would prefer). The hospital specialist palliative team discuss her concerns with her and liase with the community team so that Christine can return home. She is weak and frail. She has medication via a syringe driver and oxygen as needed. Her sister stays and friends take turns to help the family. Christine's partner cannot look after her. The district nurses attend regularly and arrange for equipment, including a hospital bed, and hospice nurses in the home for night care. The surgery reception team are made aware that any query needs prompt attention. Her usual GP visits each working day and ensures that her colleagues are aware of the situation, as not all attend the multidisciplinary meetings.

QUESTION

■ What problems might there be in communication between different professionals?

■ With shift and part-time working, there may not be continuity of care unless there is comprehensive record keeping and hand-over to others on duty.

■ There are multidisciplinary documents for end of life care to replace all other records and collate information. These are kept in the patient's home.

■ There are different patient records: the GP's, hospital records, community nursing records (likely to be kept at Christine's home), the Macmillan nurse record. If team working is well established, there should be effective communication between all parties, but information may not be passed on. Records in the patient's home aid communication, but may not be confidential and depend on everyone using them.

CASE STUDY continued

Christine's condition worsens. She was short of breath the previous night and the out-of-hours GP attended to give her some extra sedation. Her GP visits before morning surgery and liases with the district nurses and Christine's sister; they accept that she needs end of life care. This means recognising that Christine is dying, and notifying the other members of the team as well as the out-of-hours service. Christine is semi-conscious but breathing more easily. Her GP visits on her way home that evening to review and adjust any medication. She will not be working the following day. The hospice nurses can give extra medication if needed, which they do overnight after discussion with the out-of-hours GP. Christine passes away early the following morning.

QUESTION

■ What should the team do next?

The team should review Christine's case at their next meeting. Both the family and team members may need support. Some team members may have identified with Christine's age and circumstances and found the experience of looking after her more difficult than anticipated. There may be problems recognised and learning points identified for the future.

CASE STUDY: Gregory Fitzpatrick

Gregory Fitzpatrick is an 84-year-old white man who lives alone. He has asthma and in recent weeks has become increasingly frail and short of breath. He has inhalers to control his asthma but forgets to use them regularly. For a week he has been waking most nights coughing and is wheezing more on exertion. He can no longer walk to the local shops, his main contact with people in the village. He has one son living 50 miles away who is worried about his father's health and calls the GP who decides that Gregory needs an assessment but is too unwell to attend the surgery.

The GP visits Gregory at home later that day and diagnoses a chest infection exacerbating his asthma. She advises admission to hospital but he insists on staying at home. The GP is concerned about his ability to manage, so with his consent she telephones his son and then a neighbour who agrees to collect medication for Gregory. She discusses with Gregory the need for input from other professionals and back at the surgery contacts the intermediate care team, a multidisciplinary team who can attend Gregory at home. The social worker will assess his non-medical needs.

At this stage the immediate priority is to treat the acute medical problem. The GP reviews Gregory the following day and finds him improved. He agrees to blood tests and a chest X-ray. Gregory recovers well and his test results are normal. He realises that he needs help to look after himself but wants to maintain his independence at home. The social worker has already organised meals on wheels and a weekly visit to a day centre. He also requested a home assessment from the occupational therapist who can provide practical advice and equipment such as bath rails, kitchen equipment and modified seating. The physiotherapist will assess Gregory's mobility. This community rehabilitation team provide multidisciplinary support to maintain patients in the community. Usually older people become less mobile when they are unwell and may need physiotherapy to move about again with safety.

QUESTION

■ How can comunication be enhanced when professionals from different disciplines work at muliple sites?

While team meetings to review patient progress are well established in secondary care, communication between different professionals in primary care is usually less well structured. This is mainly because of greater numbers of patients seen in general practice, and the difficulty of getting all professionals together, as they may be based at a number of sites and have different work patterns. Communication and referrals between professionals in primary care are documented in patient records. GPs and practice nurses use the same records. Other community staff, for example, district nurses and physiothera-pists, use different records with copies to the GP. At the time of writing, there are some computerised links between primary and secondary care, for example, blood test results, but many hospital referral letters are paper based.

CASE STUDY continued

The GP encourages Gregory to attend the nurse-led asthma clinic scheduled for the following month. At the clinic, the nurse checks that Gregory is using his inhal-ers correctly. If his asthma control is not good, she can modify treatment.

Three months later Gregory has a fall and is found on the floor by his neighbour. He agrees to go to hospital. He is uninjured and fit for discharge a week later. However, he has to stay in hospital for a further week because of shortages of home care staff and drivers for the meals on wheels service. The hospital team (consultant, staff-nurse, physiotherapist, occupational therapists and social worker) meet prior to Gregory's discharge where they realise that Gregory cannot manage at home without these services. Information about Gregory's level of dependence at home and the adaptations he may need have been communicated to the hospital nurses via social services.

QUESTION

■ How can hospitals ensure staff work together in the most effective way to enhance the quality of care and minimise inefficencies?

Hospital teams should hold regular multiprofessional meetings where each patient on the ward is discussed. There is also a move to seven-day working in some specialities. Meetings focus on how close patients are to discharge and what their active needs are; hence what staff need to focus on that day. Meetings are an opportunity for sharing information and joint planning. Depending on how things are organised, time may be reserved for one or two patients to be discussed in depth and the patient, and often their carer, may be invited to join the meeting. Some professionals, for example, dieticians and speech and language therapists, may only be involved with a few patients so they may not attend all meetings. By having a written record of their reports or a discussion prior to meetings they can communicate their views and feed-back any decisions made.

The discussions are generally led by the nurses as they tend to have an over-view of the patient and the involvement of the family as well as any potential problems. One of the doctors will undertake the record keeping. Many teams are using multiprofessional records. The absence of information in a patient's record or the oversight of a vital piece of medical information held in another part of the health record not usually seen by a doctor, can present a very real risk of an adverse effect for a patient.

Conclusion

Health care provision in the UK is becoming increasingly complex. The two case studies in this chapter help to illustrate how doctors in primary and secondary care collaborate with other health and social care professionals to provide comprehensive and high-quality care. As well as enabling the provision of such care, interprofessional collaboration both supports doctors in their practice and enhances their professional development.

RECOMMENDED READING

- General Medical Council website, www.gmc-uk.org, and in particular *Tomorrow's Doctors Online* (2009) and *Good Medical Practice* (2006), both available on the GMC website.
- Davey P. (ed.) (2010) *Medicine at a Glance* (3ʳᵈ edn). Oxford: Wiley-Blackwell.
- Powell T. J. H. (2012) Should the UK move to graduate entry only medicine? *Student BMJ* 345: e4914.

References

Azer S. A. (2008) *Navigating Problem-Based Learning*. London: Churchill Livingstone.

Collins J. (2010) *Foundation for Excellence: An Evaluation of the Foundation Programme*. www.mee.nhs.uk/. Accessed November 2012.

DH (Department of Health) (2008) *End of Life Care Strategy: Promoting High Quality Care for All Adults at the End of Life*. www.dh.gov.uk. Accessed November 2012.

DHSSPS (Department of Health, Social Services and Public Safety) (2010) *Living Matters Dying Matters. A Palliative and End of Life Care Strategy for Adults in Northern Ireland*. www.endoflifecareforadults.nhs.uk. Accessed November 2012.

Elston M. (2009) *Women and Medicine: The Future*. London: Royal College of Physicians.

GMC (General Medical Council) (2006) *Good Medical Practice*. London: GMC.

GMC (2009) *Tomorrow's Doctors*. London: GMC.

GMC (2011) *The State of Medical Education and Practice in the UK*. London: GMC.

GMC (2012) *Leadership and Management for all Doctors*. London: GMC.

Grumbach K. and Bodenheimer T. (2004) Can health care teams improve primary care practice? *Journal of the American Medical Association* 291(10): 1246–51.

Ipsos/MORI poll (2011) *Trust in Professions*. www.ipsos-mori.com. Accessed November 2012.

King's Fund, The (2011) *Improving the Quality of Care in General Practice*. London: The King's Fund.

Ko H., Turner T., Jones C. and Hill C. (2010) Patient-held medical records for patients with chronic disease: a systematic review. *Quality and Safety in Health Care* 19: 1–7.

McLellan A., Middleton J. and Godlee F. (2012) Lansley's NHS 'reforms'. *British Medical Journal* 344: e709.

Molyneux J. (2001) Interprofessional teamworking: what makes teams work well? *Journal of Interprofessional Care* 15: 29–35.

MPS (Medical Protection Society) (2012) *The Medical Protection Society: Professional Support and Expert Advice*. www.medicalprotection.org.uk/. Accessed November 2012.

NHS (National Health Service) (2010) *The Information Centre for Health and Social Care*. www.ic.nhs.uk. Accessed May 2012.

NHS Scotland (2008) *Living and Dying Well: A National Action Plan for Palliative and End of Life Care in Scotland*. www.scotland.gov.uk. Accessed November 2012.

PMETB (Postgraduate Medical Education and Training Board) (2009) *National Training Surveys Key Findings 2008–2009*. www.gmc-uk.org. Accessed November 2012.

Vyt A. (2008) Interprofessional and transdisciplinary teamwork in health care. *Diabetes/ Metabolism Research and Reviews* **24** (Supplement 1): S106–9.

Ward L. and Innes M. (2003) Electronic medical summaries in general practice: considering the patient's contribution. *British Journal of General Practice* **53**: 293–7.

Watts G. (2012) Doctors told to collaborate with community pharmacists to improve pain management. *British Medical Journal* 344: e350.

CHAPTER 7

Midwifery

Julie Williams and Susan Davis

Introduction

Midwives and midwifery have been in existence for probably longer than any other profession identified in this book. Their history is both complex and fascinating, and provides interesting examples of interprofessional working. This is especially true in relation to medicine, and particularly to obstetrics, the medical speciality that deals with women in pregnancy and childbirth. Obstetricians and midwives have historically had the most contact and probably also the most intense interprofessional struggles, which have come to define the boundaries and the scope of midwifery and the midwife's role. It would be fair to say that there is a strong element of symbiosis between the two professions as well as some interprofessional rivalries. This chapter will chart the course of the relationship between midwifery and medicine, particularly through the last century to the present day, as an example of changing boundaries and the gradual acceptance of the need for more democratic interprofessional working.

Another concept that feeds into consideration of interprofessional working is the notion of midwifery and other health-related professions such as nursing and physiotherapy being semi-professions, rather than true professions in their own right. This was a debate that was prominent in the literature around the notion of professional status in the 1970s. It focused on the 'people working professions' or caring professions, which were, and still largely are, dominated by women. Etzioni (1969) in particular, asserted that caring professions carried lower status than professions concerned with science and ideas, and as caring was seen as an inherently female occupation, were accorded only semi-professional status. Considerable progress has been made over the past 20–30 years in raising the status of the semi-professions such as midwifery to professional status, but even today the impact this historical notion has on interprofessional working means that interprofessional communication and action may be easier with professionals such as nurses and social workers than with medical colleagues (see, for example, Murray-Davis, Marshall and Gordon 2011, Pollard 2007). Issues around the notion of professional status will therefore inform the discussion in this chapter. Much of this discussion will be carried out through the use of a case study around a pregnant woman with diabetes, which will help to identify a number of relevant issues for interprofessional working. In choosing a medically related topic, other relevant issues for interprofessional working, such as issues of neglect, domestic violence, deprivation of existing children, are excluded, but are nevertheless recognised to be of equal importance for interprofessional working.

Background and history

Midwives in the United Kingdom (UK) have a discrete role in providing care to women, their babies and families through pregnancy, childbirth and the postnatal period. They undertake this role in a variety of settings including main maternity (obstetric) units, midwifery-led units and in local communities visiting women and families in their own homes. This is not the case in many other countries, including the United States of America, where in some states midwifery is not recognised as a profession, and is even illegal. The laws that enable UK midwives registered with the Nursing and Midwifery Council (NMC) to practise are enshrined in the Nurses, Midwives and Health Visitors Act 1997 (www.legislation.gov.uk), the latest in a number of Acts that began with the Midwives Act 1902, when midwifery was first regulated as a profession (Stevens 2002). The NMC interprets the 1997 Act for practice through a series of Codes and Statements (NMC 2012a, 2012b). It also regulates and sets mandatory standards for midwives' education and training (NMC 2009). Currently, midwifery education is provided by higher education institutions and is a three-year undergraduate programme for direct entry midwives and a shorter 18-month undergraduate programme for registered adult nurses.

UK midwives recognise this framework and value the laws and education which allow them to practise legally and safely for the benefit of women and their families. Some midwives choose to opt out of the National Health Service (NHS) to go into independent practice, but are still bound by this framework. Unfortunately, independent midwifery is now under threat due to new insurance laws being introduced from the European Community (RCM 2013). Nevertheless, it is because of this legally based framework that UK midwifery is in a strong position today, able to develop and grow professionally and to work towards establishing more egalitarian relationships with the medical profession.

There has always been an uneasy relationship between midwifery and the medical profession, with the latter historically developing strategies to exclude midwifery from gaining professional status and autonomy (Witz 1992). The development of midwifery into a graduate profession has gone some way to balancing the two occupations and the emphasis on interprofessional education and working both before and after qualification has also helped considerably.

Interaction between midwifery and the medical profession is pivotal to the contemporary position of midwifery in the UK. It is important, therefore, for understanding interprofessional relationships, that some of the recent history of midwifery be explained in more depth. The relationship between midwifery and medicine came into sharper focus with the advent of 'male midwives' in the 17th century (Donnison 1988). During this period, William Smellie, a male midwife, developed his own forceps to assist women with difficult births but refused to let female midwives use them or have access to them. As a result, Smellie and other male midwives gained power over female midwives and moved into ascendancy. Medicine was developing as a profession, helped by the contemporary emphasis on rationality, the embracing of all that was considered scientific and the rejection of much that was considered folklore, old wives' tales or traditional practices. Midwives, particularly, suffered during this time, having practised traditionally for centuries, handing down unwritten wisdom from mother to daughter. These 'wise women' became marginalised and denigrated, able to offer a service only to those women too poor to pay for a doctor and subsequently increasingly lost status and recognition. All this was underpinned by the refusal of the male midwives, or obstetricians, as they were to become, to share knowledge with midwives by dint of their being female and therefore excluded from book learning. This view of women as inferior was fundamental in assigning semi-professional status to those occupations dominated by women (Witz 1992).

The history of midwifery during the latter part of the 19th century illustrates how medicine managed both to control midwifery practice and to relegate midwives to semi-professional status. During this period, a group of middle class women became increasingly concerned with the state of midwifery in England. Some doctors also wished to control midwives' practice, claiming they were ill-educated and consequently responsible for poor outcomes for mothers and babies. The efforts of both groups culminated in the Midwives Act 1902, the first Act ever to regulate UK midwifery practice (Stevens 2002). Midwives had to thereafter receive a basic training and be registered with the Central Midwives Board.

This Act proved a double-edged sword. The training received was minimal and allowed midwives to undertake duties only under the jurisdiction of doctors, to free the latter from the more tiresome aspects of their practice (Witz 1992). This was arguably the most significant act of professional exclusion that the medical profession ever exerted over midwifery; its consequences extended into the greater part of the 20th century. Davis-Floyd (2001) asserts that the Act cemented the continued unequal relationship between midwives and doctors. Doctors were given professional control over midwives' training, sat on the Central Midwives Board and examined all aspiring midwives. They effectively controlled the gateway into midwifery and this situation did not change until the Nurses, Midwives and Health Visitors Act 1979 (www.legislation.gov.uk). The 1979 Act grouped midwifery more closely with nursing and this paved the way for a different set of interprofessional relationships. These will be explored in the case study.

Professional practice

Since the mid-1990s midwifery has been a graduate entry occupation and stands on a more equal footing with obstetrics in terms of professional regard, although obstetricians and the medical profession in general continue to remain highly influential within midwifery. This is evidenced by the continued existence of two different models of maternity care and provision, the medical (or technological) model and the midwifery (or social) model. The medical model is predicated on the power accorded to the medical profession in Westernised societies. This model remains the dominant approach in mid-wifery, largely because of the major trend towards hospital-based obstetric care in the 1970s and the impact this had on reducing women's confidence in home birth and in normal midwifery care, along with increased acceptance of the medicalisation of childbirth.

This increasing medicalisation has, over the years, led to a focus on the practical and quantifiable aspects of care provision with a strong emphasis on risk assessment and reduction. Critics of this model argue that it compartmentalises and dehumanises care, with little or no attention given to psychosocial aspects, constraining women's choices within strict boundaries of what is considered to be risk-neutral (Page 2009), although this may also in part be driven by a fear of litigation. Midwives operating within this model (usually in main obstetric units) work closely with medical colleagues, engaging in interprofessional negotiation of the boundaries of professional responsibility in order to provide appropriate care to each woman. It is fair to say, however, that there is now more respect between the two professions than there has ever been and more recognition of midwives as accountable practitioners and as advocates for their clients (Murray-Davis *et al.* 2011). The stronger focus on interprofessional education has arguably made a difference to attitudes, as has the development of midwifery into a graduate profession. Professional bodies for both occupations recommend a greater level of interprofessional working and communication between midwives and obstetricians (NMC 2009, RCOG 2007). However, it is still clear that interprofessional rivalries and 'deep-seated philosophical differences over childbirth' (Reiger and Lane 2009: 320) continue to exist between midwives and doctors so work is still required to establish harmonious interprofessional relationships across the board.

The social model of care is in many ways the direct antithesis of the medical model. It aims to provide holistic woman-centred care through promoting normality in childbirth. It is critical of the risk-averse culture that surrounds the medical model, seeing this as a hindrance to the normal physiological processes supporting pregnancy and childbirth. Indeed, *Midwifery 2020* (DH 2010a) provides a blueprint for the future of midwifery and makes reference to the need to support midwifery models that encourage and facilitate normality for women and their families. Midwives who subscribe to this philosophy are likely to work within midwifery-led environments, either as community midwives or in midwifery-led birthing units. They are also more likely to want to work as independent midwives so that they can offer an even greater level of holistic woman-centred care than is available in midwifery-led units. The National

Childbirth Trust (NCT), which was established in the 1970s and has campaigned since that time for more woman and midwifery focused care, has also to a great extent influenced the move towards a social model of care. As such, this is another 'interprofessional partnership' to which the midwifery profession looks for support and engagement.

If midwifery continues to move in this direction, as encouraged by *Midwifery 2020*, interprofessional relationships will inevitably continue to change; for example, the increasing use of midwifery support workers and the changing role of midwives as they take on more technical roles. As a clear example of changing professional boundaries, the report recommends that the midwife should be the lead professional for pregnant women in most circumstances (DH 2010a). It is recommended that an obstetrician should only be the lead professional for women who have complications of pregnancy. This is a major change in professional roles since the beginning of the 1970s and represents a significant redefinition of interprofessional relationships between the two groups. Other doctors who have seen their role change as midwives assume more prominence are general practitioners (GPs), who now play a relatively secondary role in providing maternity care to their patients, mostly involving confirmation of pregnancy and some aspects of postnatal care (Wiegers 2003).

Midwifery 2020 also makes clear reference to the need for multidisciplinary working to manage the complex pregnancies that an increasing number of women experience (DH 2010a). These complexities are identified as being linked to the following factors: an increasing birth rate; an increasing number of older pregnant women, especially older first-time mothers; an increasing number of pregnancies conceived with infertility treatments; an increasing level of obesity and associated problems; and an increasing number of women surviving serious childhood illnesses, for example, cystic fibrosis. The need for effective interprofessional working is self-evident for these groups of women and so requires professionals to work together to achieve good outcomes.

Midwifery 2020 recommends that 'Women's care should be embedded in a multiagency and multi-professional arena' (DH 2010a: 26) and that there should be clear collaboration between all care providers. These care providers could include professionals such as nurses (for example, diabetic specialist nurses), medical specialists, physiotherapists and social workers, as well as obstetricians, paediatricians, anaesthetists and GPs. For communication and care to be effective, there must be respect and mutual acknowledgment of each profession's role. Murray-Davis *et al.*'s (2011) study exploring midwives' impressions of interprofessional working within one UK maternity unit, points towards some difficulties around professional hierarchies and opposing ideologies, as well as midwives being too concerned about how other professions perceive them. The authors warn that these barriers must be overcome and broader perspectives taken if multiagency and multiprofessional care is to be effectively delivered. They remain hopeful, however, that a strong focus on interprofessional education will continue to improve collaborative working in practice. It should be noted that the standards governing midwives' practice state explicitly that effective interprofessional collaboration is one of its key features (NMC 2012b).

The benefits of an empowered and strong midwifery workforce are evidenced in the narrative study conducted by Kennedy, Shannon, Chuahorm and Kravetz (2004) about midwives working from positions of strength and professional autonomy. These midwives worked with an 'engaged presence' with their clients, and drew upon their strengths to create the emotional and physical spaces to help each woman achieve a positive birth outcome. This has to be the ultimate aim for professionals involved in maternity care provision.

The White Paper *Healthy Lives and Healthy People* (DH 2011) highlights the need for partnership working between individuals and organisations. The case study that follows outlines some aspects of midwives' interprofessional working.

CASE STUDY: Emily Beech

Emily is a 30-year-old white woman in her first pregnancy and she calculates that she is about 8 weeks pregnant. She has had diabetes for 16 years. She takes insulin daily and considers her blood glucose well controlled. She has a Body Mass Index (BMI) of 28, which puts her in the overweight category, but as a diabetic, finds it difficult to control her weight. The diabetic specialist team sees her regularly and this pregnancy was planned with their support.

Ideally, any woman with diabetes planning a pregnancy should be closely monitored and known risks identified and managed before the pregnancy starts. This should include a review of her diabetes profile and diet preconceptionally by the diabetologist and the diabetic team. Blood glucose levels should be monitored every three months. Assessment of protein in the urine should also be undertaken before conception, as this gives an indication of any evidence of renal impairment; and an ophthalmologist should perform a baseline retinal examination as diabetic retinopathy can accelerate during pregnancy (Best and Chakravarthy 1997). The woman should also be advised to take nutritional supplements, especially folic acid, for three months before conception and during the pregnancy.

Preconception care is clearly vital in order to plan the pregnancy for optimal health, especially for someone like Emily, who has had diabetes for a long time. The identification of actual or potential risk factors for pregnancy by the multidisciplinary team can improve the outcome of her pregnancy and labour. Even before embarking on her pregnancy, Emily will have come into contact with a wide range of professionals, including not only the diabetic specialist team but also an ophthalmologist, ultrasonographers and dieticians. She would almost certainly have been seeing her GP, and she might have also contacted support workers in a voluntary organisation such as Diabetes UK. Her midwife may have been involved in Emily's preconception care if a joint clinic is held.

The midwife should offer Emily immediate contact with a joint antenatal and diabetes clinic (NICE 2008). In addition, the booking (first) appointment with the midwife should be carried out by the tenth week of pregnancy at the very latest. The aim of this visit is to enable Sheila (the midwife) to start to develop a relationship with Emily and her family in order to provide her with ongoing midwifery support

During the first appointment, Sheila begins to assess Emily's physical health, including her psychological and social needs, and uses the opportunity to reinforce messages about lifestyle issues that could affect the pregnancy. This approach to joined-up care is recommended by *Maternity Matters* (2007), which produced a report placing emphasis on designing individualised care for each pregnant woman. A plan of care should therefore have been drawn up and agreed by all the members of the multiprofessional team involved in providing Emily's care. The report also recommends that women and their partners should be included as members of the team, to be involved in decisions about her care and to be offered the opportunity to make their own choices where appropriate.

Sheila has an important role in providing health education and support for any changes Emily might want or need to make to her lifestyle in the light of her diabetes (Bowding and Manning 2006). Using her knowledge of local services, Sheila can work with Emily to help her make appropriate lifestyle changes.

QUESTION

■ What local voluntary or professional services might be available to provide advice and help to Emily as she seeks to make appropriate lifestyle changes?

Epidemiological studies have recommended that women with diabetes who are planning to become pregnant should be informed that effective control of blood glucose reduces the risk of miscarriage, congenital malformation, stillbirth and neonatal death (NICE 2008). Prior to becoming pregnant, Emily should have been advised by her GP and the diabetic nurse of the risks of poorly controlled blood glucose levels throughout a pregnancy but particularly during the first three months. Sheila should reinforce this advice.

QUESTION

■ What complications could occur in pregnancy, and which health professionals might need to be involved in Emily's care if they do?

The booking visit/appointment provides an opportunity for Sheila to talk to Emily about many issues related to antenatal care, including screening for abnormalities. This is particularly relevant for pregnant women with diabetes, as the risks of foetal abnormality are much increased (Yang, Cummings, O'Connell and Jangaard 2006). Sheila will measure and record Emily's height, weight and blood pressure to establish baselines for future comparison. Screening tests will be conducted during the booking visit including blood tests for anaemia, rubella, hepatitis B and syphilis along with urine tests for glucose, protein, blood and pH (acidity) level. This will assist in the process of monitoring the pregnancy and aid the early detection of potential problems. Foetal anomaly screening is recommended at

18–20 week gestation, particularly ultrasound scanning of the foetal heart (NICE 2008). The results of screening tests may lead to other, more difficult decisions, even whether or not to terminate the pregnancy. Such a situation could obviously have an adverse effect on Emily's physical or psychological health; if necessary, Sheila should offer Emily the support of a counsellor to help her and her partner, Steve, with difficult decisions.

Sheila has regular contact with Emily in order to monitor the progress of her pregnancy and to assess the health of both her and the foetus. The pattern of visits is negotiated with Emily, based on the NICE (2008) guidelines and depends upon a number of factors, including her needs as a woman with diabetes and the general progress of the pregnancy. Because of her BMI of 28 and her diabetes, Sheila identifies Emily as needing additional support. In line with the obesity guidelines (NICE 2006), Emily should be offered ongoing advice and support from a dietician about how to maintain an appropriate weight during pregnancy. Sheila therefore works collaboratively with colleagues from the wider multidisciplinary team to support Emily throughout her pregnancy.

One of a midwife's key roles is to support women's choices about the care and treatment they receive when they are pregnant (NMC 2012b). This stance accords well with the current emphasis on involving patients/service users in decision-making about their care, so that they are, in effect, bona fide members of the interprofessional team (DH 2010b). Sheila should help Emily to construct a personalised birth plan in order to enable her to feel she has as much control as possible over the birth of her baby. The birth plan is a record of Emily's choices and decisions about how she wishes childbirth to proceed and includes statements about pain relief, positions to be adopted in labour and possible interventions. Such decisions are based upon discussions between Sheila, Emily and Steve and also, because of her diabetes, the obstetrician responsible for her care. Emily will be offered induction and/or caesarean section, if indicated, when she is 38 weeks pregnant. This strategy is based on evidence that foetal death from abnormal blood glucose levels is more likely to occur after this time (Deshpande and Ward Platt 2005). If the decision is made to wait for the spontaneous onset of labour, then the midwife will undertake regular assessments of foetal well-being. This requires close cooperation and regular reporting between the obstetric, radiology and midwifery teams so is a good example of the need for effective multidisciplinary working. The birth plan forms a component of Emily's client held records and this means the professionals who attend her delivery will have access to a record of her expressed wishes.

Potential for difficulties in interprofessional collaboration may arise if Emily decides to follow a course of action during her pregnancy which conflicts with medical or midwifery advice. In such a situation, Sheila is professionally obliged to act as an advocate for Emily, that is, to support her in her choices and to communicate with other relevant professionals (NMC 2012b); this may require Sheila to exercise high-level negotiation skills (see Chapter 2) as many other professionals do not have a similar obligation of advocacy with respect to their patients.

As part of collaborative working, the midwife has a responsibility to liaise with and inform the local health visitor of Emily's pregnancy as (s)he may wish to make a home visit when Emily is 34 weeks pregnant. This will help the health visitor to provide continued support when Sheila ceases professional contact with Emily. Under normal circumstances, a woman and her baby are discharged from midwifery care between 10 and 28 days after birth, but in some cases the midwife continues to be involved and works in partnership with the health visitor. This may well be the case for Emily who may need additional support if she experiences complications at or after the baby's birth. The health visitor will have a responsibility to monitor the progress and well-being of Emily's baby from 14 days until 5 years.

CASE STUDY continued

During her pregnancy it is important for Emily to keep her blood glucose levels within the recommended normal range. Her targets are set in a joint diabetic clinic with the obstetrician and diabetologist taking into account the risks of abnormal blood glucose levels for the foetus. In addition, Emily is advised to check her blood glucose level one hour after every meal.

Emily feels this is a chore and does not always do it, but she does test her blood glucose levels nightly before going to bed. On one occasion, she adjusts her rapid-acting insulin and this results in her blood glucose level falling very quickly. Steve wakes in the night and finds Emily unconscious. He cannot rouse her and calls the paramedic team. Emily is treated at home by the paramedics, but because of her pregnancy she is admitted to the antenatal ward for observation and stabilisation of her blood glucose levels.

QUESTION

■ What professionals would have been involved in this event and what would their role be?

Support is given by other health professionals in the accident and emergency department. Midwifery care would also have been provided during this incident should Emily have been subsequently admitted to the hospital's maternity unit for closer observation.

CASE STUDY continued

The pregnancy continues without further incident. An anaesthetic assessment is offered during the final three months of pregnancy and Emily and her partner are advised of the care following delivery if she needs general anaesthesia. Because of the possibility of an emergency caesarean section, the anaesthetist and the theatre team are kept informed of Emily's progress during labour. Baby Willow is eventually born at 38 weeks following induction of labour and a normal delivery. A hospital-based midwife looks after Emily during labour, so she meets another member of the midwifery team at this time. This midwife is guided by the birth plan written by Emily in conjunction with Steve, Sheila and the obstetrician caring for her during her pregnancy.

Consistent with NICE (2008) recommendations, Willow remains with Emily on the postnatal ward where the midwives require knowledge of Emily's pregnancy, labour and diabetic status in order to provide both mother and baby with appropriate care. Appropriate care is always predicated on effective communication within the interprofessional team and is vital for quality patient care. When Sheila visits the ward four hours later, a midwife is testing Willow's blood glucose level as part of the observation of clinical signs for neonatal complications. This is in line with the recommendations for the care of the baby of a mother with diabetes (NICE 2008). Willow is feeding well and is monitored by a midwife or paediatrician for her feeding pattern and any potential abnormalities in her blood glucose levels developing during the first 24 hours after her birth.

Conclusion

The midwife's role encompasses all aspects of pregnancy and childbirth and, while it is possible for a midwife to work in isolation, women's expectations and the continued existence of vulnerable groups make it imperative that midwives develop their potential to work interprofessionally with a range of professionals who may provide support to pregnant woman and new mothers. The changing relationship between obstetricians and midwives continues to support more effective collaborative working than in the past. Additionally, the increase in complex pregnancies requires that all professionals involved in maternity care work collaboratively. The case of Emily provides an example of how midwives can work collaboratively with other professionals as they aim for the best outcomes for both mothers and babies.

RECOMMENDED READING

- Billington M. and Stevenson M. (2007) *Critical Care in Childbearing for Midwives*. Oxford: Blackwell.
- Downe S., Byrom S. and Simpson L. (2011) *Essential Midwifery Practice: Leadership, Expertise and Collaborative Working*. Chichester: Wiley-Blackwell.
- Downe S., Finlayson K. and Fleming A. (2010) Creating a collaborative culture in maternity care. *Journal of Midwifery and Women's Health* **55**(3): 250–4.
- Jones L. and Bennett C.L. (2012) *Leadership in Health and Social Care: An Introduction for Emerging Leaders*. Banbury: Lantern.

References

Best R.M. and Chakravarthy U. (1997) Diabetic retinopathy in pregnancy. *British Journal of Ophthalmology* 81(3): 249–51.

Bowding J. and Manning V. (2006) *Health Promotion in Midwifery: Principles and Practice* (2nd edn). London: Hodders Arnold.

Davis-Floyd R. (2001) Daughters of time: the shifting identities of contemporary midwives. *Medical Anthropology* 20: 105–39.

Deshpande S. and Ward Platt M. (2005) The investigation and management of neonatal hypoglycaemia. *Seminars in Foetal and Neonatal Medicine* 10: 351–61.

DH (Department of Health) (2010a) *Midwifery 2020: Core Role of the Midwife: Workstream Final Report*. London: DH.

DH (2010b) *Equity and Excellence: Liberating the NHS*. Norwich: The Stationery Office.

DH (2011) *Healthy Lives and Healthy People*. White Paper. London: DH.

Donnison J. (1988) *Midwives and Medical Men: A History of the Struggle for Control of Childbirth* (2nd edn). London: Heinemann.

Etzioni A. (1969) *The Semi-Professions and their Organisation: Teachers, Nurses and Social Workers*. New York: Free Press.

Kennedy H.P., Shannon M.T., Chuahorm R.N. and Kravetz M.K. (2004) The landscape of caring for women: a narrative study of midwifery practice. *Journal of Midwifery and Women's Health* **49**(1): 14–23.

Maternity Matters (2007) *Maternity Matters: Choice, Access and Continuity of Care in a Safe Service*. London: DH.

Murray-Davis B., Marshall M. and Gordon F. (2011) What do midwives think about interprofessional working and learning? *Midwifery* **27**: 376–81.

NICE (National Institute for Health and Clinical Excellence) (2006) *Obesity: Guidance on the Prevention, Identification, Assessment and Management of Overweight and Obesity in Adults and Children* (modified 2010). London: DH.

NICE (2008) *Diabetes in Pregnancy: Management of Diabetes and its Complications from Pre-Conception to the Postnatal Period*. London: DH.

NMC (Nursing and Midwifery Council) (2009) *Standards of Proficiency for Pre-Registration Midwifery Education*. London: NMC.

NMC (2012a) *The Code: Standards of Conduct, Performance and Ethics for Nurses and Midwives*. London: NMC.

NMC (2012b) *Midwives Rules and Standards*. London: NMC.

Page L. (2009) Woman-centred, midwife-friendly care: principles, patterns and culture of practice. In Fraser D. and Cooper M. (eds) *Myles Textbook for Midwives* (15th edn). London: Churchill Livingstone.

Pollard K. (2007) Discourses of unity and division: a study of interprofessional working among midwives in an English NHS maternity unit. PhD thesis. http://eprints.uwe.ac.uk. Accessed July 2013.

RCM (Royal College of Midwives) (2013) *Independent Midwives and Medical Malpractice Insurance*. www.rcm.org.uk. Accessed June 2013.

RCOG (Royal College of Obstetricians and Gynaecologists) (2007) *Safer Childbirth: Minimum Standards for the Organisation and Delivery of Care in Labour*. London: RCOG.

Reiger M. and Lane L. (2009). Working together: collaboration between midwives and doctors in public hospitals. *Australian Health Review* **33**(2): 315–24.

Stevens R. (2002) The Midwives Act 1902: An historical landmark. *Find all citations in this journal (default)*.

Orfilter your current search

RCM Midwives **5**(11): 370–1.

Wiegers T. (2003) General practitioners and their role in maternity care. *Health Policy* **66**(1): 51–9.

Witz A. (1992) *Professions and Patriarchy*. London: Routledge.

Yang J., Cummings E.A., O'Connell C. and Jangaard K. (2006) Foetal and neonatal outcomes of diabetic pregnancies. *Journal of Obstetrics and Gynaecology* **108**(3 part 1): 644–50.

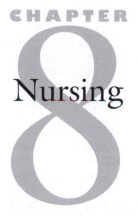

CHAPTER
8
Nursing

Derek Sellman, Matthew Godsell and Mervyn Townley

Introduction

In the United Kingdom (UK) the title 'registered nurse' can be used only by someone whose name is on the national register of nurses held by the Nursing and Midwifery Council (NMC). Each of the four recognised fields of nursing (adult nursing, children's nursing, learning disabilities nursing, and mental health nursing) claims a particular specialist area of practice and each has its own section of the NMC register.

Students of nursing undertake a three-year full-time (or equivalent) course of study in preparation for registration and subsequent practice as a nurse. The three-year course comprises 2300 hours of practice and 2300 hours of theory. The NMC require that nurses 'be able to provide essential care to anyone while also delivering specialist care in one of the four fields of practice' (NMC 2010: 9). Preregistration nursing courses have been delivered within higher education institutions since the diploma of higher education became the standard level of academic preparation during the 1990s and the move to all degree preparation programmes was completed in September 2013. Following successful completion of a preregistration nursing programme and successful application for admission to the NMC register, a qualified nurse can be employed in professional nursing work where they are required to develop their knowledge and skills as part of continuing professional development linked to maintaining active registration.

At the point of registration a nurse becomes accountable for her or his own practice. The nature of this professional accountability has been a debate of some significance since at least the 1980s and reflects what some consider to be an emerging sophistication in nurses' perceptions of themselves as autonomous and professional care givers. Nurses have struggled to define the nature of nursing and as a consequence there are a number of competing defintions within the literature. Thus, while many believe nursing to be merely a matter of common knowledge, just what that supposed common knowledge actually is has continued to defy articulation. This is to say that while everybody thinks they know what nurses do, a formal universally accepted definition of nursing remains elusive.

This is partly because there is so much variation in what nurses do in providing care that spans the full range between the emotional and the social as well as the physical. In addition to the four fields of nursing there are numerous nursing roles including: research nurses, school nurses, community nurses, consultant nurses, nurse teachers, public health nurses, nurse managers, infection control nurses, chemotherapy nurses, and so on. What each of these types of nurses actually does can be so different that it is difficult to encapsulate a single idea of the nurse.

One commonly cited definition of nursing is:

> The unique function of the nurse is to assist the individual, sick or well, in the performance of those activities contributing to health or its recovery (or to a peaceful death) that he would perform unaided if he had the necessary strength, will or knowledge. And to do this in such a way as to help him gain independence as rapidly as possible.
>
> (Henderson 1966: 15)

A more recent definition developed by the Royal College of Nursing (RCN) and used by the NMC to inform the development of the 2010 *Standards for Pre-registration Nursing Education* states that nursing is:

> The use of clinical judgement in the provision of care to enable people to improve, maintain, or recover health, to cope with health problems, and to achieve the best possible quality of life, whatever their disease or disability, until death.
>
> (RCN 2003: 3)

That these two definitions span a period of nearly 40 years illustrates that effort continues to be expended on the attempt to define nursing and indicates that the task remains one of complexity. It is not the purpose of this chapter to attempt a definition of nursing nor to provide a definitive account of what nurses do. Rather the aim is to provide a snapshot of some professional nursing activity within the context of interprofessional working.

While it is true that nursing is a universal activity performed by trained and untrained individuals in both voluntary and paid capacities, this chapter is concerned with the work of professional nurses working in the UK in the early part of the 21st century. It should be recognised that the work of nurses is not exclusive to registered nurses; many others provide nursing care within and outside of the formal organisation of care delivery. In hospital and community settings some aspects of nursing are provided by unregistered health care workers (albeit under the supervision of registered nurses) who may have undertaken some training and education. But a great deal of nursing care is provided on a voluntary basis by friends, family and others in the community. As discussed in Chapter 3, the importance of the role of these carers and the significance of their contribution to health and social care should not be underestimated.

In addition, the boundaries that separate the four fields of nursing are not always easy to distinguish. Patients, after all, do not necessarily fit neatly into one of the four categories. Both adults and children may have learning disabilities and/or suffer mental health difficulties as well as a requirement for nursing care for physical illnesses or the promotion of positive health.

Among nurses there is a continuing debate about the proper term that should be used to describe those who are in receipt of professional nursing. Nurses who work in acute areas of practice tend to use the term 'patient', those working with people with learning disabilities tend to consider 'service user' to be the appropriate term, 'clients' is the term often employed by mental health nurses, and 'children' or 'young people' appear to be terms preferred by children's nurses. It is possible that each term reflects a set of political or ideological beliefs about the nature of persons, the nature of health and the nature of health care such that it might be claimed that 'patient' indicates a passive role; that 'client' suggests a more active relationship; and that 'service user' indicates some form of egalitarian partnership. If the choice of term does reflect a difference of perspective then the potential for tension between nurses from different fields of practice needs to be acknowledged lest it gets in the way of effective collaboration. In the nursing literature it is not unusual to see the phrase 'patient or client', or 'patient/client'. Such language can be cumbersome and confusing. For this reason 'patient', 'client', and 'service user' will be used as interchangeable terms throughout this chapter representing nothing other than a description of someone in receipt of nursing practice.

To outline some of the complexities of nursing the material in this chapter is presented in two sections. In section one the case of Frank, a man with moderate learning disabilities who has suffered a heart attack, offers an insight into the roles of both adult and learning disabilities nurses. Section two outlines the child and adolescent mental health services using the case of Theresa to illustrate some aspects of the work of both children's and mental health nurses. In the first scenario, staff are drawn together in response to the needs of a particular individual; in the second scenario, it is staff already working in an established interprofessional team who respond to the person's needs. Thus the two case studies offer contrasting approaches to team work and collaboration.

Section 1: Adult and learning disabilities nursing

CASE STUDY: Frank Burton

Frank Burton has been transferred from a coronary care unit following an acute myocardial infarction (heart attack). He is a 45-year-old man with moderate learning disabilities. Frank seems to understand the content of most everyday conversations but does not appear to comprehend the information he has been given about his heart condition. His ability to convey thoughts, feelings and ideas using full sentences is limited. When he was admitted to the medical ward he attempted to make his needs, likes and dislikes known using a combination of single words, facial expressions and pointing but found it very difficult to make himself understood and now he appears to have given up trying to communicate directly with either the staff or the other patients. He is friendly and will often smile and maintain eye contact when people approach him but he does not attempt to move beyond this stage towards a more significant relationship. He relies on his mother, Julie, to communicate with the team. Similarly the staff have come to rely on Julie and sometimes they seem reluctant to engage with Frank unless she is present. Julie feels that the doctors and nurses are happy to talk to her about some things, for example the sort of things that Frank likes to eat or drink, but they do not involve her or Frank in any significant discussions about his health. She thinks that being in an unfamiliar environment, combined with Frank's shyness and his restricted vocabulary, has made him feel isolated and uncomfortable. She is concerned about his well-being because she knows that he does not like to make a fuss and will conceal anxiety, discomfort and pain rather than draw attention to himself.

Nursing care for Frank

Following the acute phase of Frank's time in hospital his care plan will be reviewed in the light of his changing needs now that he has been transferred to the medical ward. It is particularly important for the nurses to monitor and record Frank's blood pressure and pulse as well as the electrical activity of his heart (he may continue to be attached to a cardiac monitor and will have a 12-lead electrocardiogram (ECG) recorded regularly). These observations provide an indication of his cardiac recovery and help to determine the most appropriate stage of his rehabilitation. The nurses will also aim to ensure Frank remains pain free and can breathe easily so that he can undertake the recommended amount of physical activity. Although Frank has been given advice about what he should or should not do, the doctors and nurses that have spoken with him suspect that he has not understood or retained what he has been told. Julie has stated that she does not believe that he has grasped the significance of his illness. She is concerned that he is attempting to do too much because he thinks that he will be able to go home sooner if the staff see him doing more for himself. Julie is also worried about the care that people with learning disabilities receive in hospital. She has read two Mencap publications (Mencap 2007, 2012) and the report produced by the Parliamentary and Health Service Ombudsman and Local Government Ombudsman (PHSO&LGO 2009). These documents do not present a positive image of general hospital care for people with learning disabilities.

The findings reported by Sir Jonathan Michael show that Frank and Julie's experiences are not unusual. The report states that (outside specialised services that are specifically for people with learning disabilities):

> There is insufficient attention given to making reasonable adjustments to support the delivery of equal treatment, as required by the Disability Discrimination Act. Adjustments are not always made to allow for communication problems, difficulty in understanding (cognitive impairment), or the anxieties and preferences of individuals concerning their treatment.
>
> (DH 2008: 7)

The report has also indicated that Julie's situation is not exceptional:

> Parents and carers of adults and children with learning disabilities often find their opinions and assessments ignored by healthcare professionals, even though they often have the best information about, and understanding of, the people they support. They struggle to be accepted as effective partners in care by those involved in providing general healthcare; their complaints are not heard; they are expected to do too much of the care that should be provided by the health system and are often required to provide beyond their personal resources.
>
> (DH 2008: 7)

The evidence produced by Mencap (2007, 2012) and the Parliamentary and Health Service Ombudsman and Local Government Ombudsman (PHSO&LGO 2009) has shown that the relationship between Frank and his mother and the ways in which they relate to the staff will be a key factor in determining the success of Frank's treatment. If Julie felt that her opinions were valued then she might develop a closer relationship with the team on the ward and this might encourage Frank to attempt to disclose more to the team. Similarly if members of the team were able to approach Frank in a more confident manner, and were not so dependent on Julie, they might strengthen their relationship and develop more effective ways of working with him.

QUESTIONS

- Consider who might be included in the interprofessional team caring for Frank.
- How could different members of the interprofessional team make improvements to Frank's care and improve the quality of care for other people with learning disabilities that will be admitted to the ward?

Did you think of Julie and Frank as integral members of the team? The nurses might want to make Julie feel that her contributions are valued by spending some time with her and seeking her opinions. This could mean that one person in the team will assume responsibility for making the relationship stronger. It would not mean that the team was committed to accepting everything that Julie suggested. The team might make more effort to acknowledge that she knows Frank best and explore ways of using Julie's knowledge to improve his care. For example, Julie can draw their attention to specific aspects of Frank's non-verbal communication because she is used to reading and interpreting his behaviour every day.

Did you identify a role for a speech and language therapist? A speech and language therapist could work as a member of the team to help devise ways of improving communication with Frank. This might involve augmenting his speech using pictures or symbols to convey his likes, dislikes and needs. A useful source for symbols is The Noun Project (www.thenounproject.com) which aims to build a global repository of universal symbols. The speech and language therapist might also be able to work as part of the team to develop the presentation of information in a format accessible to people with learning disabilities.

Did you mention a liaison nurse? The role of the acute liaison nurse was described in the Michael Report as providing health facilitation or link working 'between and across primary and secondary specialised (acute hospital) care' (DH 2008: 41). Liaison nurses might improve the service that a person going into hospital will receive by visiting the individual at home prior to admission to learn about his or her likes, dislikes, strengths and needs. They can arrange for the individual to visit the ward prior to admission so that she or he can see what it is like and will have some idea about what to expect. Liaison nurses might also work with staff on the ward to develop and implement a plan that will meet the individual needs of a patient with learning disabilities.

An essential feature of cardiac rehabilitation is the need to help patients recognise the risk of further cardiac problems and how to avoid them. David, Frank's primary ward nurse, has been discussing Frank's care with Ishani, a student nurse in the second week of her allocation to the ward. During the conversation David referred to the importance of health promotion and they discussed the role that nurses play in educating patients and promoting healthier lifestyles. He told her that on this ward they use a standard approach to health promotion that involves providing patients with written information and then checking that they understand which lifestyle changes will reduce the likelihood of further heart attacks. David and Ishani recognised that the standard approach would not work with Frank. In her last study block Ishani had gone to a lecture about improving the standards of care for people with learning disabilities. She remembered that the lecturer mentioned a communication passport and she told David that a passport would have helped them to make adjustments to Frank's care plan so that it was more likely to meet his needs. A passport is a document that a patient takes into hospital and that provides essential information about likes and dislikes as well as about strengths and needs. It might contain, for example, details about how the person communicates, information on medication, fears and phobias and so on. In this respect, it can assist all members of the interprofessional team as they interact with a patient.

David has set Ishani some learning objectives to achieve during her placement that involve locating and summarising guidance on improving the experience of people with learning disabilities in acute settings. Ishani contacted the liaison nurse to ask for advice; the liaison nurse suggested that she and Ishani work together and with the rest of the ward team. She also recommended that in order to meet her learning objectives Ishani read the RCN dignity document (RCN 2010) that has particular relevance to the care of people with learning disabilities when they are receiving health care. Ishani read the document and referred to the notes she had made during the last study block. Using this information she produced a list of action points.

QUESTIONS

■ What could you do to make an immediate improvement in Frank's care?
■ How would you make improvements over a longer period?

Ishani said that she would spend time during her shifts getting to know Julie. She said that she would ask Julie how members of the team might gain a more reliable impression of Frank's feelings and how they might make better judgements about the extent of his understanding. She also thought that the following points from the RCN provided useful guidance for everyone that had regular contact with Frank:

■ every time something new is introduced explain what is happening and why
■ [explain] who everyone is, what they do and why they are there – in ward round situations, minimise the amount of staff present and ensure everyone is introduced to the person
■ [talk about] what's going to happen afterwards
■ [describe] who gets to see the relevant information

(RCN 2010: 6).

David agreed that maintaining regular contact with key people would be good for Frank. He told Ishani that they should try to maintain the balance between Frank's comfort and recovery by drawing upon the full range of professionals that might be in a position to assist Frank. They both recognised it would be impractical to try to restrict the number of different individual practitioners involved in his care but they thought they might be able to facilitate collaborative practice among the various professionals by constructing a plan that would encourage each of them to approach Frank in a consistent way. For example, by using appropriate forms of communication and spending a bit more time talking to him, trying to explore some of the things he finds difficult to understand.

Ishani thought that the communication passport was a good idea. It might contain pictures or photographs accompanying key words related to things he wanted/did not want from the team (images that conveyed his preferences; for example, his preference for a cold rather than a hot drink, or for tea rather than coffee) and his feelings (images that would convey when he felt tired or upset or in pain). Her lecture notes referred to a passage on assessing pain:

> Tools do exist to assist staff in assessing the pain of disabled patients who cannot communicate verbally. Such tools, used in conjunction with family carers'

knowledge and appropriate training, can be used to prevent unnecessary pain. Every member of staff whose role involves pain treatment needs to be aware of the potential difficulties in diagnosing pain in patients with a learning disability. This is especially important in cases that involve people with limited verbal communication

(Mencap 2012: 15)

Ishani thought that the team should make assessing Frank's pain and discomfort their immediate priority. She also made a note to ask the liaison nurse for any 'easy read' leaflets about heart attacks, healthy eating and healthier lifestyles. The important characteristics of easy-to-read material include plain English, large fonts so that there are not too many words on a single page, and plenty of illustrations/photographs. Although Frank may not be able to read and understand all of the printed information on the leaflets they would be the starting point for a discussion and they might encourage practitioners to sit down and talk with him about the content.

David and Ishani also thought about forward planning and how they might make the most effective use of the resources that were available within the hospital. They identified Julie as the most useful source of information about Frank and they wanted to involve her in assembling material for a passport that Frank would identify as his own. In addition to her knowledge, she might contribute photographs that could be used as objects of reference. David and Ishani also made a list of professionals that were likely to be involved in his ongoing care. The list included the liaison nurse who would have useful contacts in the community learning disabilities team nearest to Frank's home and his general practitioner. They also thought about preparing a discharge sheet following guidance provided by the RCN (2006) to contain information in an accessible format covering Frank's diagnosis, treatment, follow up appointments, medications and their side effects as well as the name of a contact person from the ward in case Frank or Julie require any additional information. Each of these actions would reflect a commitment to interprofessional working beyond the hospital and into the community, representing an essential aspect of collaboration between primary and secondary care.

Section 2: Child and adolescent mental health services

This section provides an outline of the role of nurses who work in child and adolescent mental health services (CAMHS). CAMHS brings together skills identified in two fields of nursing: children's nursing and mental health nursing. It is not possible in a short chapter of this type to explore in detail the differences between the two fields of nursing but it should be noted that nurses who work in CAMHS can be registered under different parts of the NMC register. While the majority of CAMHS nurses are registered under the mental health section of the register, there are a significant number who are registered as children's nurses. The respective preregistration courses equip nurses with different but complementary skills that contribute to effective interprofessional working in CAMHS. Throughout the UK CAMHS is organised in different ways as a result of both local service development and reorganisation attempts to offer a coherent service in any given region. The Health Advisory Service Report (HAS 1995) describes CAMHS as a four-tiered system of care and this continues to be the model on which service provision is based in the UK (HIS 2011). The four tiers represent different levels of service provision which become more specialist in order to respond to more intense and complex problems or disorders. Professionals employed at tier one, or primary care, (for example general practitioners, school nurses and teachers) are not employed with skills in providing specialist child mental health care. Therefore, when they come across more complex problems, they will need to refer clients to specialist services such as: the generic specialist practitioners at tier two; the more intense specialist teams and day units at tier three; or the highly specialised services such as inpatient units at tier four.

At tier one a range of nurses may be involved in the promotion of mental health for children. Most of the work at this stage is likely to be health promotion or simple strategies that do not require specialist training in children's mental health. By way of an example, school nurses may be involved in sex education, advice and guidance about aspects of bullying, recognition of specific mental health problems, and teaching stress reduction strategies to children.

There is evidence of considerable mental health problems and disorders in children and young people with an estimated 2–5 per cent of children seen in primary care settings having mental health problems as their main complaint (Spender, Salt, Dawkins *et al.* 2001); and according to the Department of Health 'One in ten children aged between 5 and 16 years has a mental health problem' (DH 2011: 8). On the basis of these figures, it would appear that significant numbers of children and young people will come to the attention of different professionals working in tier one services. When more specialised help is required referrals can be made to one or more of the other three tiers of CAMHS. The introduction of the primary mental health care worker (who might come from a number of professional groups but is often a nurse) has been a response to the recognition of a need to bridge the gap between the services at tiers one and two.

Those working in tier two services include professionals who are trained specifically in assessment and management of children and young people with mental health problems. Professionals in tier two services work alongside other CAMHS professionals to undertake formal assessment of clients and work with other, non-CAMHS, professionals to offer advice and to suggest appropriate therapeutic interventions.

Tier three and four services usually provide specialist services for children and adolescents with mental health problems and disorders. Tier three involves professional teams working collaboratively to provide services while tier four provides highly specialised services in the form of intensive packages of care including: inpatient facilities, eating disorder teams, and secure units usually on a regional basis. Nurses who are part of CAMHS specialist teams will have completed some form of post-registration education in children and young persons' mental health. It is the specialist services provided in tiers three and four that will be the focus of the remainder of this section.

The specialist services of tiers three and four are organised in different ways and located in different settings in different parts of the UK. In some areas tier three community teams are based on the same site as tier four inpatient units and, in some cases, close working relationships have developed between the two. In others areas there may be as many as five or six services based in different locations, all with small teams of different professionals with inpatient and day patient services organised as separately managed units. Some of the professionals in these small teams will liaise with professionals of the same background in the other teams – others may not. This variation in the configuration of CAMHS has been a cause of concern in a number of reports (CAMHS review 2008, HAS 1995, NAW 2001).

Although there is concern about some aspects of the variation in service provision there remains a recognition of the need for flexibility in order to meet local and national mental health needs of young people. The specialist CAMHS teams may be based in small general hospital sites, children's hospitals, health centres or may be housed in purpose-built premises. Most teams will have at least one nurse although there are some teams without nurses. Under existing salary structures there is a belief that nurses represent value for money and consequently form the largest professional group in the specialist services (CSM 2009/10, Joughin, Jarrett and Maclean-Steel 1999). In the continuing era of financial constraints this has become an increasingly important consideration.

Children and young people who are referred to the specialist services present with a range of difficulties including: eating disorders; mood disorders; severe anxiety; hyperactivity; and various behavioural problems. Although any illness in a child is likely to create anxiety for parents this is particularly marked with issues that relate to mental health. There remains stigma and ignorance around mental health problems and disorders (Thornicroft 2006) and this can make it especially difficult for children and young people as well as for their parents. For nurses and other professionals one of the most challenging aspects arising from this area of work is to engage children and young people, and their families with the range of therapeutic activities on offer. Parents can feel that they have failed in some way in their parenting role and this may result in conflict with CAMHS professionals. One of the most important roles that nurses may find themselves required to fulfil is to help parents develop strategies to deal with the complex problems and needs of their children. This may mean running specific parent training programmes such as the *Webster-Stratton* training programme (Webster-Stratton 2011) or the *Three P's* programme (Boyle, Sanders, Luzker *et al.* 2010).

As well as specific therapeutic skills for different situations there are a number of recurring themes that nurses working in CAMHS need to recognise as important. There have been some well-documented cases, including the cases of Victoria Climbié and Baby P, highlighting the need for effective child protection measures to be in place across agencies. Corby (2000) notes that there is a high correlation between child abuse and mental health problems and it is now widely accepted that communication between agencies is essential. Nurses working within CAMHS are therefore required to develop the skills to recognise abuse, act appropriately using local procedures, and be able to communicate effectively with other professionals as part of interprofessional working with various agencies (DH 2007).

Children and young people who make use of CAMHS may be of any age between 4 and 18. In tier four services, day and inpatient treatment units tend to distinguish between, and work separately with, children (usually taken to include 4- to 11-year-olds) and adolescents (12–18). However, following the lead from other countries such as Australia and the USA there are moves to develop youth mental health services which typically cater for young people aged 16–23 years. Other, sessional type, services based in clinics typically work with children and young people across the age range. This requires that nurses, like other professionals, be flexible in the therapeutic approaches used. Parental consent is required for all treatment approaches with young children but if adolescents/young people are competent to give consent, as determined by using the Fraser guidelines (Brazier 2003), there is no formal requirement for parental consent. The issue of consent for treatment raises a related issue of confidentiality. Nurses are required to 'uphold the standards of their professional code' (NMC 2008: 1) and this means that, in the case of a competent young person, the young person's permission is necessary before the release of her or his confidential information. This can create difficulties for nurses working with young people who experience problems in their relationship with their parents. Parents often ask for information about what their child is saying or doing in therapy sessions and sometimes become angry and frustrated when told that this is confidential. This is a particularly sensitive area and one in which many nurses become skilled. Of course, there are limits to this confidentiality especially where information is revealed in relation to child protection issues or illegal activities. And just as it is for all nurses, CAMHS nurses need to ensure their clients understand the limitations of the confidential nature of the therapeutic relationship.

Issues of interprofessional working in CAMHS

Inpatient units are typically staffed by a nursing team in order to provide cover for the 24-hour period while day units tend to be staffed during normal office hours. There is no nationally agreed formula for the configuration of nursing staff so the skill mix across the UK varies considerably. Indeed the background of CAMHS nurses also varies insofar as there may be any combination of children's, adult, learning disability, and mental health nurses in post, although the majority of nurses working in CAMHS have a mental health qualification. In addition there may be other professionals such as occupational therapists, teachers (who provide statutory education services), play therapists, social workers, psychologists, psychotherapists and psychiatrists. Some teams remain influenced by the view that the consultant psychiatrist is the natural leader of the multidisciplinary team and consequently has the most power and control in decision making. This hierarchy, which perhaps reflects a medical rather than social model of health and health care, is challenged in some teams where nurses (or other team members) exert a strong influence. Tensions sometimes arise in the relationships between nurses and other team members (especially medical staff) as a result of these sorts of dynamics. In the inpatient units nurses provide care for the full 24-hour period while other professionals work more traditional sessional hours (usually 09.00–17.00). These working practices need careful management in order to provide young people with the maximum benefit to be gained from the range of skills and approaches of each professional. One of the most important themes to arise in these environments is the need for consistency of approach to care. Effective communication is considered to be essential in the provision of a consistent service to children and young people with mental health problems and disorders.

Similar issues can arise in CAMHS teams based in clinics and/or community settings. Such teams are also made up of a range of different professionals including nurses. A typical team might comprise two nurses, a consultant psychiatrist, a psychologist, a social worker, a family therapist and a play therapist. CAMHS teams seem to function best where the professional background of each team member is utilised to meet specific needs of clients and where the traditional hierarchy and power relationships have been eroded. Indeed, current strategies (CAMHS review 2008, DH 2003, NAW 2001) support the development of non-hierarchical teams in recommending that CAMHS should aim for clear and effective ways of interprofessional working.

The skills of CAMHS nurses

From all that has been said so far it can be seen that nurses make up a significant part of the professional workforce offering services to children and young people with mental health problems or disorders. Individual nurses often develop specific therapeutic skills and collectively there is a wide range of different skills and knowledge among nurses working in CAMHS. This would typically include: core counselling skills; a range of therapeutic approaches such as cognitive behavioural therapy, dialectic behavioural therapy, motivational interviewing and solution focused therapy; knowledge of child development; an understanding of parenting skills; and working in teams to assess risk factors and recognise stress and distress in relationships.

Following Townley's (2002) recommendations, children's mental health issues have been incorporated into the curriculum for preregistration training in the UK although the amount of time spent on this in the curriculum varies considerably. Nevertheless, many of the skills learnt as part of preregistration education for children's or mental health nursing are relevant and readily transferable to the CAMHS environment. In addition, once working in CAMHS, nurses often take the opportunity to develop more specialist skills by accessing post-registration education. Such courses are designed to provide nurses with appropriate knowledge and skills and would include courses in family therapy, cognitive behavioural therapy, psychotherapy, group work, as well as more specific courses for working with certain client groups such as those with eating disorders or attention deficit hyperactivity disorder. Much of the post-registration training is available to a range of different professionals and one of the strengths of shared learning is the development of a greater understanding of the differences in cultures and roles.

From this brief overview it should be apparent that CAMHS offers a complex range of services from a number of different professionals with various backgrounds. The way in which these professionals interact can vary enormously depending on where the service is, how the team is configured and, of course, the individual personalities and experiences of each professional. The following case study of a young person referred to a tier three CAMHS team is used to illustrate some of these complexities.

CASE STUDY: Theresa

Theresa is a 15-year-old girl admitted to a general hospital children's unit following an overdose of paracetamol tablets. She has revealed that she has recently self-harmed by cutting her arms and she has several scars as a result.

This particular children's unit employs a nurse to liaise between the ward and CAMHS; a role similar to that of the primary mental health care worker. As such she is able to offer advice, support and supervision to the ward nurses who, generally speaking, lack experience of children's mental health problems, and she acts as a link between the two services. It is envisaged that the primary mental health care worker will undertake a similar role by liaising with the primary care services. One of the advantages of a liaison nurse is that she is in a position to make a risk assessment once the routine medical assessment has been completed. There is evidence to suggest that nurses and other health and social care professionals have negative attitudes towards young people who self-harm (Bywaters and Rolfe 2002). The liaison nurse can help to reduce the stigma associated with mental health problems in children and young people and this can be of enormous benefit to both staff and the young people themselves.

The normal process for this particular CAMHS team requires a written referral which is then considered against agreed criteria at the weekly team meeting. Although not an emergency service, in this case and because of the concerns of the liaison nurse, the team agreed to visit Theresa before receiving a written referral. The consultant psychiatrist made the first visit because she is one of only a few members of the team with the authority to prescribe medication. From the information provided the team believed Theresa might need to be prescribed antidepressant drugs although this would not normally be the first treatment approach even in such cases.

CASE STUDY continued

Following assessment by the consultant psychiatrist it was thought Theresa was not clinically depressed and therefore did not require a course of antidepressant medication. However, it was clear she was experiencing some emotional turmoil in several aspects of her life including in her relationships with her mother and her boyfriend as well as some difficulties in school. Self-harm seemed to be her way of coping.

The team believed they could offer support to Theresa, monitor her mood and provide some therapeutic interventions in relation to her self-harming behaviour. Each of these entail therapeutic approaches that could be provided by several members of the team. Sanura, a nurse, was the one CAMHS team member with specific experience of working with clients such as Theresa and because Sanura had both the expertise and the capacity to take on a new client she became Theresa's key worker.

It is important that the needs and interests of a client are taken into account when choosing the most appropriate professional to engage in therapy with the client. However, this can have the effect of reducing the exposure of other team members to working with certain client groups and, as a result, some team members may miss opportunities to develop particular skills. In some instances the decision about which team member is to be the primary worker for a given client is a pragmatic one. That is, it may need to be whoever is available and has the time to accept another client. There are sometimes long waiting lists for CAMHS and consequently some team members with particular skills are in such demand that they simply may not have the capacity to meet the needs of clients with urgent or emergency needs in the timeframe required. In Wales, for example, health targets to address this require children to be seen within 16 weeks although in some areas the introduction of the Choice and Partnership Approach (CAPA) has reduced this considerably (York and Kingsbury 2009).

Options for the most appropriate place for Sanura to meet with Theresa include: in the family home, in the clinic setting, at school, or in a neutral setting such as a local cafe. In some cases it is helpful to meet the child with her or his parents and in other instances it is appropriate to meet with the whole family. On some occasions there may be a need for two professionals from CAMHS to meet with the family or child. One underlying principle in deciding when and how to meet with a child or young person is that her or his wishes and needs should be taken into account. In this case Sanura and Theresa agree to meet in the clinic.

During the course of Sanura's counselling work with Theresa it became known that six months previously she had been hit on the back of the head by her father. All professionals in CAMHS undertake training in child protection and all services are required to have child protection procedures in place. Good practice entails exploring what confidentiality means at the beginning of any therapeutic process and Theresa had been informed that if she or any other child was thought to be at risk from harm or had been harmed then this would need to be reported. The assessment of risk in these kinds of situations is complex (Quinney, Thomas and Whittington 2009) and requires expert advice. Thus, Sunara contacted the local authority social services department duty officer who noted that this was not an emergency child protection situation because the reported hitting had occurred several months earlier. As a result Sanura knew that a discussion of the issues could wait until the next scheduled weekly team meeting. At the meeting it was felt that the parents should be asked to meet with someone from the team to discuss parenting strategies with a specific remit to ensure that the risk to Theresa of being hit again might be reduced. If one therapist undertakes therapeutic interventions with different individuals from the same family there is always the possibility of a conflict of interest. For this reason the team came to the view that it was important that Sanura should not be involved in the work with the parents as this could affect her therapeutic relationship with Theresa. Following discussion the team recognised that the social worker within the CAHMS team was the most appropriate team member to work with Theresa's parents because of his experience and expertise in child protection issues. This work involved two sessions during which Theresa's parents were invited to explore parenting strategies and issues related, in particular, to the setting of boundaries of acceptable behaviour for Theresa in order to reduce the likelihood of harm to Theresa.

CASE STUDY continued

Sanura's work with Theresa lasted for a number of months and as a result she learned to manage her feelings in more constructive ways and this reduced her tendency to self-harm. She would talk to friends about her feelings and she recognised the need to remove herself from situations when she began to feel angry. She also learned to talk with her parents, which resulted in more realistic expectations on the part of Theresa and her parents. Theresa did not stop self-harming altogether but did recognise the need to take more control of her situation.

Counselling was the most appropriate intervention with Theresa but other therapeutic approaches may be used by CAMHS professionals depending on the individual needs of the client. For some clients family therapy is perceived to be the appropriate form of work. Many nurses and other professionals working in CAMHS have experience of working with families as units and some have formal training as family therapists. Although not always possible, it is common to do this work with two professionals as this provides two perspectives on family dynamics and enables support and supervision for team members.

Some clients benefit from pharmacological therapy. Young people who suffer from clinical depression can be helped by the use of antidepressant drugs after other therapeutic approaches have been exhausted or deemed unsuitable and other examples include: the use of medication where a young person has a psychosis, suffers from attention deficit hyperactivity disorder, or has a severe anxiety state. As a general principle, medication will only be prescribed for young people where there is evidence for its likely effectiveness. Where medication is prescribed, one part of the role of a CAMHS nurse is to help monitor the effectiveness of medication on the young person.

Some young people experience mental health problems as a result of illegal drug use and CAMHS team members may well liaise with a local substance use service if it is felt to be of therapeutic value to a particular client. Part of the role of a CAMHS nurse is to be able to both recognise when there is a need to link with other services and to know how to access those other services.

This requires knowledge and understanding of appropriate services from which CAMHS clients might benefit.

Conclusion

This chapter has offered an insight into the nature of some aspects of the work of the four fields of nursing, together with examples of interprofessional working. Individual nurses work in different settings using different sets of skills but share a common goal of providing a comprehensive service tailored to meeting the nursing needs of each patient. The recognition that a service can only meet all the health and social care needs of people if nurses work collaboratively with other professionals is beginning to make a real difference to nursing practice.

RECOMMENDED READING

- Broussine E. and Scarborough K. (2012) *Supporting People with Learning Disabilities in Health and Social Care*. London: Sage.
- Dogra N., Parkin A., Gale F. and Clay F. (2009) *A Multidisciplinary Handbook of Child and Adolescent Mental Health for Front-line Professionals* (2nd edn). London: Jessica Kingsley.
- Sellman D. and Snelling P. (eds) (2010) *Becoming a Nurse: A Textbook for Professional Practice*. Harlow: Pearson.

References

Boyle C.L., Sanders M.R., Luzker J.R., Prinz R.J., Shapiro C. and Whitaker D.J. (2010) An analysis of training, generalization, and maintenance effects of Primary Care Triple P for parents of pre-school-aged children with disruptive behavior. *Child Psychiatry and Human Development* **41**(1): 114–31.

Brazier M. (2003) *Medicine Patients and the Law* (3rd edn). Harmondsworth: Penguin.

Bywaters P. and Rolfe A. (2002) *Look beyond the Scars*. London: NCH.

CAMHS Review (2008) *Children and Young People in Mind: The Final Report of the National CAMHS Review*. www.nationalarchives.gov.uk. Accessed June 2013.

Corby B. (2000) *Child Abuse: Towards a Knowledge Base* (2nd edn). Buckingham: Oxford University Press.

CSM (Children's Mapping Services) (2009/10) *CAMHS National Workforce Summary*. www.childrensmapping.org.uk .Accessed June 2013.

DH (Department of Health) (2003) *Getting the Right Start: National Service Frameworks for Children – Emerging Findings*. London: DH.

DH (2007) National Service Framework for Children Young People and Maternity Service: The mental health and psychological well-being of children and young people: Standard 9. www.nationalarchives.gov.uk. Accessed June 2013.

DH (2008) *Healthcare for All: Report of the Independent Inquiry into Access to Healthcare for People with Learning Disabilities (The Michael Report)*. www.dh.gov.uk. Accessed April 2012.

DH (2011) *No Health without Mental Health: A Cross-government Mental Health Outcomes Strategy for People of All Ages*. www.gov.uk. Accessed June 2013.

HAS (Health Advisory Service) (1995) *Child and Adolescent Mental Health Services: Together We Stand*. London: HMSO.

Henderson V. (1966) *The Nature of Nursing: A Definition and its Implications for Practice, Research, and Education*. New York: Macmillan.

HIS (Healthcare Improvement Scotland) (2011) *Integrated Care Pathways for Child and Adolescent Mental Health Services: Final Standards.* www.healthcareimprovementscotland.org. Accessed June 2013.

Joughin C., Jarrett L. and Maclean-Steel K. (1999) *Focus on Who's Who in Child and Adolescent Mental Health Services.* London: Royal College of Psychiatrists' Research Unit.

Mencap (2007) *Death by Indifference.* www.mencap.org.uk. Accessed April 2012.

Mencap (2012) *Death by Indifference: 74 and Counting.* www.mencap.org.uk. Accessed April 2012.

NAW (National Assembly for Wales) (2001) *Child and Adolescent Mental Health Services Everybody's Business.* Cardiff: NAW.

NMC (Nursing and Midwifery Council) (2008) *The Code: Standards of Conduct, Performance and Ethics for Nurses and Midwives.* www.nmc-uk.org. Accessed February 2012.

NMC (2010) *Pre-registration Nursing Education in the UK.* www.nmc-uk.org. Accessed February 2012.

PHSO&LGO (The Parliament and Health Service Ombudsman and Local Government Ombudsman) (2009) Ombudsman's report calls for urgent review of health and social care for people with learning disabilities. www.ombudsman.org.uk. Accessed April 2012.

Quinney A., Thomas J. and Whittington C. (2009) *Working Together to Assess Needs, Strengths and Risks.* www.scie.org.uk. Accessed December 2012.

RCN (Royal College of Nursing) (2003) *Defining Nursing.* London: RCN.

RCN (2006) *Meeting the Health Needs of People with Learning Disabilities: Guidance for Nursing Staff.* London: RCN.

RCN (2010) *Dignity in Health Care for People with Learning Disabilities.* London: RCN.

Spender Q., Salt N., Dawkins J., Kendrick T. and Hill P. (2001) *Child Mental Health in Primary Care.* Oxford: Radcliffe Medical Press.

Townley M (2002) Mental health needs of children and young people. *Nursing Standard* 16(30): 38–45.

Thornicroft G. (2006) *Ignorance + Prejudice + Discrimination = Stigma.* London: Mental Health Foundation.

Webster-Stratton C. (2011) *The Incredible Years: Parents, Teachers, and Children Training Series: Program Content, Methods, Research and Dissemination, 1980–2011.* Seattle: Incredible Years Inc.

York A. and Kingsbury S. (2009) *The Choice and Partnership Approach – A Guide to CAPA.* Bournemouth: CARIC Press in association with S & G Group Ltd.

9

Occupational Therapy

Fiona M. Douglas and Helen Martin

Introduction

Occupational therapists work in both health and social care environments focusing on the extent to which service users are able to carry out day-to-day activities, or occupations. The list of activities that most people do, and take for granted, includes such seemingly simple tasks as putting out the rubbish, brushing teeth, and washing or ironing clothes. Other things that individuals do which are especially meaningful might include, for example, making a meal for family or friends, walking the dog, playing with children or grandchildren, and repairing the car. These lists merely illustrate the importance of ordinary activities in contributing to meaningful patterns of daily life that make us who we are; and it is these activities that make up our occupations (Kramer, Hinojosa and Royeen 2003, Wilcock 1998). The work of occupational therapists involves assisting individuals in the pursuit of their everyday occupations. Usually this assistance is needed when an individual's capacity to pursue their occupations is compromised in some way.

Origins

Occupational therapy is a relatively new profession with origins in the 19th century movement pressing for moral treatment of the insane (Peloquin 1989). In 1917 this approach to mental health care was adopted by the National Society for the Promotion of Occupational Therapy which later became the American Occupational Therapy Association (Christiansen and Baum 1997). The six people credited with founding occupational therapy as a profession are: William Rush Dunton – a psychiatrist; George Edward Barton – an architect; Eleanor Clarke Slagle – an almoner/social worker; Susan Cox Johnson – a teacher of arts and crafts; Susan Tracy – a nurse; and Thomas Bessell Kidner – another architect. They shared a common belief in the merits of occupation as therapy and their different professional backgrounds illustrate the diversity from which occupational therapy originated and which continues to influence current practice.

In Britain elements of occupational therapy were in evidence following the first world war with the rise in demand for rehabilitation services. However, the development of the profession in the UK began towards the end of the 1920s with the opening of the first occupational therapy clinic (Allendall Clinic) in 1929 and the first occupational therapy training school (Dorset House) in 1930, both in Bristol (Wilcock 2002).

The nature of occupation

While the term occupation is often used to describe the type of paid employment people undertake, for occupational therapists, occupation is defined as everyday, routine and personally meaningful activities. We say that someone is occupied when they are engaged with a task and this illustrates a recognition of the wider general meaning of occupation. In the early part of the 20th century, when the profession was founded, this general meaning of the term occupation described any activity that kept a person busy. It was selected by the founders as a term broad enough to encompass all aspects of the activity of people.

Many things influence our occupations, not only what we do but also the way in which we do them. Cultural, family and social aspects of our lives, as well as the physical environment, are perhaps the most obvious influences on our occupations. This means that our occupations are uniquely individual, although influenced by culture, learning and environments (Zemke and Clark 1996).

Becoming an occupational therapist

To become an occupational therapist requires graduate level study and once qualified, an occupational therapist must be registered with the Health and Care Professions Council (HCPC) in order to practise anywhere in the UK. There are more than 20 university-based undergraduate pre-registration programmes in the UK, each registered with the World Federation of Occupational Therapists (WFOT). WFOT status ensures comparable standards and means graduates are eligible for state registration in any WFOT affiliated country. In the UK, pre-registration programmes for occupational therapy are currently validated jointly by the HCPC and the College of Occupational Therapists.

The idea that people are occupational beings, or that people need to be engaged in activities, is fundamental to the concept and the practice of occupational therapy. The assumption is that doing meaningful things is necessary for the well-being of the individual and provides opportunities for both health and personal choices. The work of occupational therapists is therefore an attempt to enable individuals to engage in meaningful occupation. This requires a perspective that recognises the uniqueness of each person whose well-being is best served by matching occupation to ability without limiting that person's capacity to meet challenges. As a result, occupational therapists consider partnership working to be essential (Law, Baum and Baptiste 2002) and this partnership includes working with both service users and carers as well as with different health and social care professionals. Occupational therapists work in interprofessional teams with almost any combination of, among others, nurses, physiotherapists, homecare workers, equipment service personnel, social workers, speech and language therapists, doctors, clinical psychologists, community care workers, music therapists, teachers, architects, builders and surveyors.

Occupational therapists work in many different areas but wherever employed will follow the occupational therapy process of assessment, planning of intervention, implementation of intervention and evaluation of intervention (Finlay 2004). This process begins with the occupational therapist developing an intentional therapeutic relationship (Taylor 2008) demonstrating the ability to adapt their approach and behaviour to best benefit the person with whom they are working. This flexibility may be referred to as the therapeutic use of self (Hagedorn 2001, Martin and Wheatley 2008).

Regardless of the challenges to a person's occupations, the focus of the occupational therapist is on the impact of those challenges on the person's occupational performance. Assessment is undertaken initially through discussion with the person and whoever knows them well. The central elements are:

- The person's day-to-day *routines* – past ones, what they are doing at present and what they hope to do in the future
- The person's various *roles* – past, present and hoped for
- Which *occupations* have *supported* the person's well-being – especially those they enjoy
- Considering any *occupational deprivation or limited participation* due to the person's current situation and their inability to engage in all their *occupations*.

The following case studies illustrate the role of the occupational therapist working within interprofessional teams.

CASE STUDY: Maud Gilbert

Maud Gilbert is a 91-year-old widow who lives alone in a warden-supported flat. Following a fall at home, she was admitted to the medical assessment unit where the staff includes doctors, general nurses, a mental health nurse, physiotherapists, occupational therapists, social workers, dieticians, pharmacists and generic support workers.

On admission, Maud was found to be malnourished and exhibiting signs of confusion in relation to time and place. Prior to admission she was able to get around her flat using a walking frame, and used her shopping trolley as a walking aid outside. Her mobility on the unit is restricted as her balance is poor and her eyesight limited. Despite appearing confused, she is pleasant and cooperative. She is very private, having lived on her own since her husband died 28 years ago. She has two sisters, but because of their own particular circumstances, neither feels able to offer Maud any practical support. Maud says she does not have any friends and appears to have little social interaction. Her daughter, Sylvia, who lives a few miles away, holds Maud's chequebook, does most of her shopping and manages her laundry. Sylvia reports that her mother has been showing signs of urinary and faecal incontinence. She is not sure that Maud can safely return home, noting that her mother has recently reported not knowing where she is, has phoned during the night to say she had just returned from a walk and what a nice day it is, and has been saying 'odd' things such as she used to live in Scotland and had recently had a dishwasher installed (neither being true). Although registered blind, Maud does have residual vision and likes to do crosswords and other types of puzzles; she also likes to listen to music. She does not like watching television and does not own one.

QUESTION

■ What factors are important for the occupational therapist to consider when approaching Maud?

As Maud has shown some signs of confusion, is in a strange environment and has recently sustained a fall, she may be frightened and anxious. Therefore it is vital that the occupational therapist approaches her in a sensitive but encouraging and supportive way to enable the development of a positive relationship. As Maud has limited vision, the first meeting should occur in a room with a good natural light source, as this may help her to see the occupational therapist and to read her facial expression and body language. The occupational therapist might also arrange a first meeting with Maud when her daughter can be present so that she can offer reassurance. This will also help encourage a positive and trusting working relationship to be formed between the occupational therapist, Maud and Sylvia, as all parties will know what has been said.

QUESTION

■ What questions do you think the occupational therapist might ask Maud and her daughter?

The occupational therapist will ask questions designed to elicit information about Maud's occupations pertinent to any interventions needed to assist Maud in her current situation. The aim of questioning will be to discover something about Maud's likes and dislikes, her capacities and incapacities, and her needs and desires. Questions that would help the occupational therapist in these aims could include:

■ Can you tell me about your usual daily routine?
■ Do you have breakfast before getting dressed?
■ What do you like to eat for breakfast?

- Do you cook lunch or an evening meal?
- Do you have any daily or weekly chores?
- Do you go out during the week or monthly?
- What do you enjoy doing in your daily routine?
- What do you hope to be able to do in the future?
- What is really important to you?
- Do you have any grandchildren with whom you would like to keep in touch?
- What weekly activities would you like to maintain?
- What are some of the things that you miss being able to do?

The occupational therapist will ask Maud these questions, but Sylvia may also contribute information and help build a picture of the things that Maud likes to do, things she can do, things she would like to do more and/or other things she might like to do. The answers to these questions will also assist the occupational therapist to assess Maud's current functional ability as well as her safety in engaging in meaningful and important occupations.

For example, following a first meeting with Maud and Sylvia, Kelly (the occupational therapist) discovers that Maud's preferred breakfast is a poached egg. However, she hasn't attempted to cook one for months because she finds it difficult to judge how much water to put in the pan and to see when the water is boiling. Instead, her breakfast has consisted of tea and toast which may have contributed to her malnourishment. Kelly suggests that Maud tries microwaving poached eggs instead and both she and Sylvia seem keen to explore this option. Kelly will then arrange for Maud to come to the occupational therapy department kitchen to be observed making a cup of tea and poaching an egg in the microwave. Before the visit, Kelly will try to replicate Maud's home kitchen as much as possible so that she can accurately assess her ability to manage once transferred home. Kelly will share the outcome of her assessment of Maud's abilities in the kitchen with those members of the interprofessional team most involved in decision making regarding Maud's future care. That is, in particular, doctors, ward nursing staff, the physiotherapist and the social worker as this will help to ensure that any package of care will be based on Maud's assessed needs. For example, if Maud cannot manage to poach an egg in the microwave, or struggles with toasting bread safely, then Maud and Sylvia together with the interprofessional team might consider it best to have carers go in twice a day to help her prepare her meals. Alternatively, Maud could have a weekly delivery of meals that could be stored in her freezer.

Other aspects of the occupational therapy assessment will include Maud's ability to: manage her money; get washed and dressed; safely negotiate her way around her flat; and continue to engage with her favourite activities.

Managing her money

Sylvia has reported that Maud seems to have difficulty recognising coins and notes, and has told her that when she buys her morning paper she hands over notes as she cannot see the value of the coins in her purse. Sylvia is worried that this makes her mother vulnerable. Sylvia has now applied for Power of Attorney to handle Maud's affairs.

In England someone can choose to appoint Powers of Attorney in advance, where they nominate one or more persons to make decisions on their behalf regarding finances and/or their health and welfare should they become unable to do this for themselves. This is a legal process that, under the Mental Capacity Act 2005 (www.legislation.gov.uk), offers protection to those lacking the capacity to make decisions for themselves. The person with Power of Attorney is required to involve the person in whose interest they are acting as much as possible in any decisions made, and must always consider which choices would benefit them most.

Washing and dressing

Kelly will also assess Maud's ability to wash and dress herself safely. She will liaise with the unit staff regarding a suitable date to undertake this assessment. It is important that it occurs during the morning at the time Maud usually does these things in order to reinforce her orientation in time. The nurses have been encouraging Maud to wear continence pads but she often forgets to put these in place. Kelly can help by placing the pads in Maud's underwear drawer as a visual prompt towards establishing a routine of putting on a pad in the morning while getting dressed.

Getting around her flat

As Maud was unable to account for the fall at home that resulted in her admission, Kelly may accompany Maud on a visit to her flat to assess her functional ability in her home environment. Kelly would be looking for environmental hazards that can be rectified relatively easily with Maud's approval, such as the removal of loose rugs. There are many simple changes that can make a home environment much safer for someone in Maud's situation. Examples include: raising the height of chairs or the bed using chair or bed raisers, installing a raised toilet seat, and adding a toilet frame or grab rails to make transfers easier. It is likely, if Maud is in agreement, that Sylvia and other appropriate members of the interprofessional team, such as the home warden, will be invited to attend the home assessment.

Engaging with enjoyable activities

Kelly could also offer advice in terms of Maud's leisure occupations. It might be, for example, that Maud would find it helpful to use a magnifying glass or magnifying sheet when completing her puzzles, or it might help to make minor adjustments to the positioning or brightness of room lighting.

QUESTION

■ How do you think the occupational therapists role contributes to interprofessional care?

Working as part of the interprofessional team, the information gathered by Kelly will contribute to Maud's overall assessment in relation to whether or not she can be transferred safely home to her flat. The interprofessional team will likely include doctors, nurses, physiotherapists and social workers. In this instance the focus of the interprofessional team is to enable a safe discharge for Maud. The doctors and nurses will lead the assessment of her physical health ensuring she is medically stable, the physiotherapist will focus on Maud's mobility and muscular strength, and Kelly will be assessing her functional ability and independence to manage safely at home. The social worker may be involved in setting up a package of care for transfer home that may involve some day care assistance, such as the weekly delivery of frozen meals and a carer visiting to cook these for Maud, or attendance at a day care facility if this is what she would like. The social worker may also work with Maud's daughter to explore her needs and entitlements as a carer.

Other members of the interprofessional team who may be involved with Maud include: speech and language therapists, continence advisor, dieticians (who may suggest appropriate dietary supplements), pharmacists, ward clerks, discharge liaison staff, the community mental health team for older people, the general practitioner (GP), the warden of her block of flats, volunteers with links to other services, and the intermediate care team (if it is deemed that Maud would benefit from a short period of intensive rehabilitation).

CASE STUDY: Kim Miles

Kim Miles is a 28-year-old single mother diagnosed with bipolar disorder 5 years ago. She has an 18-month-old son, Geoffrey, who lives with Kim's mother and stepfather about 5 miles away. This arrangement was agreed at a multiprofessional meeting as being in Geoffrey's best interests given Kim's inability to care for her son adequately on her own. At the same meeting a child protection plan (DfE 2013) was developed to ensure Geoffrey's safety.

QUESTION

- Who do you think would have been involved in developing this plan?

In England and Wales, the Department for Education has overall responsibility for child protection and issues guidelines that local authorities use to produce their own policies and procedures to guide practice in child protection. In developing the child protection plan for Geoffrey it is likely that doctors, health visitors, social workers, Kim, Kim's mother and stepfather, and her community psychiatric nurse would have been present. The plan has provision for Kim to visit Geoffrey once a week. Kim often needs to be reminded to visit and is usually accompanied by a member of the community mental health team. During the visits Kim plays with Geoffrey for only a few minutes before leaving. This angers Kim's mother and frustrates her stepfather who blames Kim for making life difficult for them.

Kim leads a somewhat chaotic lifestyle. She lives in a one-bedroom housing association flat that she says she likes. The local housing association works in partnership with the community mental health team to provide guaranteed-for-life accommodation for vulnerable single people in a bid to bring some stability to their lives. The flat is very untidy. Kim leaves clothes on the floor and dishes unwashed in the kitchen. She does not appear distressed by this although she does become frustrated when she cannot find things she is looking for. However, she shows no inclination to start tidying her flat or to sort out items.

Kim enjoys taking short walks in the surrounding countryside as well as shopping for clothes, although once she brings her purchases home, they often remain unopened. She likes cooking and shopping for food but will purchase ingredients without first checking what she already has in her cupboards, so it is not unusual to find, for example, three pots of mustard or four packets of unopened spaghetti in her kitchen. The oldest items tend to be pushed towards the back of the cupboards but she sees this as normal and displays no desire to tidy her cupboards.

Kim drives and enjoys the freedom this affords her, often undertaking long journeys without telling anyone she is going away. She recently joined an Internet dating agency and has arranged to meet men after brief exchanges of details; she seems unaware of the potential dangers inherent in this. Twice in the last month she has driven over 100 miles to meet men first contacted in this way only to return home within a few days upset that the relationship disintegrated so quickly. On both occasions she forgot to take her medication with her.

Kim is under the care of an Assertive Outreach Team, a specialised team available seven days a week that works with those service users with severe mental health challenges who find it hard to engage with appropriate mental health care services (Firn 2007). Assertive Outreach Teams take services to the service users' environment, be it their home or a cafe, for example, and aim to encourage a positive and beneficial working relationship through flexible arrangements. The teams try to ensure frequent meetings and maintain a high level of flexibility and will, among other things, accompany service users to appointments or help them engage in important and meaningful activities.

The Assertive Outreach Team working with Kim consists of community psychiatric nurses, mental health support workers, social workers, occupational therapists and mental health workers. Kim's key worker has been a community psychiatric nurse but Kim's engagement with the team remains sporadic, often being out when they call for pre-arranged appointments. Kim's medication is prescribed by her GP but she often forgets to take it. Currently, a mental health support worker calls at the flat daily to remind Kim to take her medication but sometimes she is not at home.

The interprofessional team have decided that closer involvement with an occupational therapist might help Kim add some structure to her life and help her to develop her skills of independent living. It is therefore agreed that Bernadette (the occupational therapist in the team) will take on the role of Kim's key worker.

━━━━━━━━━━━━━━━━━━━━ **QUESTION** ━━━━━━━━━━━━━━━━━━━━

■ What do you think will be the role of the occupational therapist when working with Kim?

Bernadette, an experienced occupational therapist, has agreed to take a lead in working with Kim. Bernadette understands the requirement of a long-term commitment and knows to expect setbacks as well as successes. Much of Bernadette's work will involve establishing a relationship of trust, finding out what Kim considers to be her most important and meaningful occupations, and then collaborating with Kim to agree an intervention plan on which they can work. Bernadette knows that she will need to remain flexible and adaptable if she is to first gain and then retain Kim's trust during the next few months. The skills that Bernadette will need while working with Kim will include: using her occupational therapy problem-solving approach; remaining open, approachable and non-judgemental; maintaining a calm and relaxed approach; aiming for partnership working practices with Kim; and retaining a positive 'can-do' outlook (Duncan 2011, Hughes 2008). By utilising these skills Bernadette will be able to help Kim work towards achieving her desired goals.

Building a relationship might start in any number of ways but Bernadette begins by calling in for coffee as an unrushed way of getting to know Kim. After a few visits to the flat, Bernadette accompanies Kim on a couple of shopping trips. This helps to build the relationship of trust further because shopping is something that Kim likes to do and she experiences their time together as enjoyable.

Once Kim regards the relationship as non-threatening, Bernadette suggests that they visit Geoffrey together. Kim likes this idea and when they arrive at her parents' house, Bernadette takes the opportunity to model appropriate engagement with Geoffrey while encouraging Kim to behave likewise. Bernadette praises Kim's interest in her child and encourages Kim to stay and play with him a little longer on each visit. Bernadette recognises that in this way it might be possible to help Kim build a stronger routine of meaningful visits to her son.

Kim responds positively to the visits to her son and begins to enjoy Geoffrey's company, much to the delight of Kim's mother and stepfather. Not every visit is a success but Kim has started to look forward to seeing her son on a regular basis. Inspired by this progress, Bernadette slowly begins to work with Kim on building other structured activities and occupations. For example, they work together on developing a regular weekly shopping and cooking routine. Working in a stepwise fashion, Bernadette starts with merely accompanying Kim when she shops for food before encouraging her to decide on a menu before buying food. Bernadette can then build on this routine by helping Kim to check the food already in her cupboards before writing a shopping list. In this way Bernadette helps Kim to plan her meals as well as organise her cupboards, things that can help to reduce the chaos in her life. There will, of course, be successes as well as setbacks and a balance with the things that Kim enjoys needs to be maintained. To this end Bernadette might build on other things that Kim enjoys such as going for walks, which could be extended into Kim taking her son for a walk in his stroller.

In all this, Bernadette will have demonstrated the use of profession specific skills of activity analysis to identify the life skills Kim needs to develop in order to achieve what she desires. Specialist skills are defined by the College of Occupational Therapists as 'the expert knowledge and abilities that are shared by all occupational therapists, irrespective of their field or level of practice' (COT 2009: 4). They will then agree upon small achievable steps to work towards as interim measures (Creek 2003). This specialist skill is referred to by occupational therapists as *grading* (Ormston 2002). The steps need to give Kim something achievable to work towards so that she will experience success to help maintain motivation. If Kim is able to progress with this it is likely that other daily and weekly occupations could be addressed such as doing laundry on a weekly basis and aspects of housework on a daily basis. It is likely to take several months for Kim to embed new routines into her daily living.

Bernadette will also be able to help Kim explore any long-term aspirations she might have. If, for example, Kim thinks she might like eventually to find paid employment then this will depend on many factors including the local employment situation and available services. There might be a local vocational rehabilitation service that already employs occupational therapists to help people with mental health problems and/or learning disabilities to find volunteering opportunities, work experience, or paid employment. Other staff working in vocational rehabilitation services can include physiotherapists, psychologists, disability employment advisors, case managers, Job Centre Plus Personal Advisers and Employment Support Workers. It is possible that Kim would consider voluntary work as a start in developing a work routine.

QUESTION

- Who else would the occupational therapist need to liaise with?

Team working provides myriad opportunities for collaboration and Bernadette may need to liaise not only with Kim, Kim's parents and Geoffrey's social worker, but also with community nurses, mental health workers within the Assertive Outreach Team, and the GP. With Kim, Bernadette will undertake the intervention planning and design, although it will probably be a mental health support worker who will perform some of the day-to-day work of the plan. Thus it is important for the team to build a number of trusting relationships with Kim, communicate clearly with her about their work, keep up-to-date records, and use forms of language that everyone understands. It might be, for example, that on the days Bernadette visits, she will take responsibility for reminding Kim to take her medication. Effective communication here would entail ensuring that the mental health support worker knows she need not visit on those days. As is often the case, community teams work flexibly and with some overlap between roles (Molyneux 2001) although team members do bring their profession-specific skills to their work. This is important because effective interprofessional teams and systems of communication are key to avoiding unnecessary duplication of effort.

Conclusion

Occupational therapists focus on day-to-day meaningful occupations that give routine and shape to a person's life. Disruptions to daily routine caused by, for example, illness or the consequences of a serious accident, can prevent someone carrying out meaningful activities and can lead to a de-skilling, a feeling of uselessness and, in extreme situations, a loss of self-identity. Through working in close partnership with the person, identifying with them the form their daily life takes, their preferences for doing tasks and their present capacities, an occupational therapist can enable them to try out different ways of engaging with their occupational tasks.

Working as part of an interprofessional team, an occupational therapist carefully analyses the components of the task or occupation and tries to match those to the person's present capacities. The expertise of the occupational therapist lies in getting just the right amount of challenge in the task so that the person will experience a sense of achievement. This becomes the person's motivation to succeed in regaining skill, which in turn reactivates a sense of purpose and self-identity.

In the case studies presented in this chapter, Maud and Kim can be seen to have experienced disruptions in their daily occupations and in different ways an occupational therapist was able to assist them to re-establish meaningful occupations. These occupational therapists worked collaboratively within interprofessional teams with shared goals for the service users, with mutual understanding of how these would be achieved and with an endorsement of each team member's skill, knowledge and professional values. In so doing the occupational therapist contributed a valuable set of skills and perspective to the service-user and the interprofessional team.

RECOMMENDED READING

▤ College of Occupational Therapists, www.cot.co.uk.

▤ Creek J. and Lawson-Porter A. (2007) *Contemporary Issues in Occupational Therapy Reasoning and Reflection.* West Sussex: John Wiley & Sons.

▤ Duncan E. (2012) *Foundations for Practice in Occupational Therapy* (5th edn). Toronto: Churchill Livingstone Elsevier.

▤ Kielhofner G. (2009) *Conceptual Foundations of Occupational Therapy Practice* (4th edn). Philadelphia: F.A. Davis.

▤ Mackenzie A., Craik C., Tempest S., Cordingley K., Buckingham I. and Hale S. (2007) Interprofessional learning in practice: the student experience. *British Journal of Occupational Therapy* [online] **70**(8): 358–61.

References

Christiansen C.H. and Baum C.M. (eds) (1997) *Occupational Therapy: Enabling Function and Well-being* (2nd edn). New Jersey: Slack.

COT (College of Occupational Therapists) (2009) *Definitions and Core Skills for Occupational Therapy*. www.cot.org.uk. Accessed February 2012.

Creek J. (2003) *Occupational Therapy Defined as a Complex Intervention*. London: COT.

DfE (Department of Education) (2013) *Working Together to Safeguard Children*. www.education.gov.uk. Accessed January 2014.

Duncan E.A.S. (2011) Skills and processes in occupational therapy. In Duncan E.A.S. (ed.) *Foundations for Practice in Occupational Therapy* (5th edn). Toronto: Churchill Livingstone Elsevier, pp. 33–42.

Finlay L. (2004) *The Practice of Psychosocial Occupational Therapy* (3rd edn). Cheltenham: Nelson Thornes.

Firn M. (2007) Assertive outreach. *Science Direct* **6**(8): 329–32.

Hagedorn R. (2001) *A Structured Approach to Core Skills and Processes*. Edinburgh: Churchill Livingstone.

Hughes S. (2008) Approaches to severe and enduring mental illness. In Creek J. and Lougher L. (eds) *Occupational Therapy and Mental Health* (4th edn). Edinburgh: Churchill Livingstone Elsevier, pp. 409–24.

Kramer P., Hinojosa J. and Royeen C.B. (eds) (2003) *Perspectives in Human Occupation: Participation in Life*. Baltimore, MD: Lippincott Williams and Wilkins.

Law M., Baum C. and Baptiste S. (2002) *Occupation-Based Practice: Fostering Performance and Participation*. New Jersey: Slack.

Martin M. and Wheatley S. (2008) The developing student practitioner. In Creek J. and Lougher L. (eds) *Occupational Therapy and Mental Health* (4th edn). Philadelphia: Churchill Livingstone, pp. 237–50.

Molyneux J. (2001) Interprofessional teamworking: what makes teams work well? *Journal of Interprofessional Care* **15**(1): 29–35.

Ormston C. (2002) Roles and settings. In Creek J. and Lougher L. (eds) *Occupational Therapy and Mental Health* (4th edn). Philadelphia: Churchill Livingstone, pp. 213–36.

Peloquin S. (1989) Moral treatment: contexts considered. *American Journal of Occupational Therapy* **43**: 537–44.

Taylor R.R. (2008) *The Intentional Relationship*. Philadelphia: F.A. Davis.

Wilcock A.A. (1998) *An Occupational Perspective on Health*. New Jersey: Slack.

Wilcock A.A. (2002) *Occupation for Health: A Journey from Self-health to Prescription, Vol. 2*. London: British Association and College of Occupational Therapists.

Zemke R. and Clark F. (1996) *Occupational Science: The Evolving Discipline*. Philadelphia: F.A. Davis.

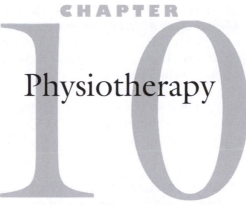

Physiotherapy

Dianne Rees

Introduction

This chapter provides an overview of the physiotherapy profession in the United Kingdom (UK), including its scope of practice and potential career pathways. Key factors in relation to pre-qualifying education and continuing professional development are presented. A case study is used as a vehicle for exploring one area of physiotherapy practice in more detail (neurology physiotherapy). This also allows exploration of interprofessional working in a specialist environment (a stroke unit) where effective team work is an essential component of patient care. The chapter concludes with some 'food for thought' on the potential direction of the physiotherapy profession in the future.

Scope of practice and regulation

Physiotherapy is:

> a health care profession concerned with human function and movement and maximising potential. It uses physical approaches to promote, maintain and restore physical, psychological and social well being, taking account of variations in health status.

> (CSP 2002: 19)

The scope of physiotherapy practice is broad and complex and physiotherapists have traditionally used a wide variety of physical means to treat patients.

Manual techniques (such as complex joint mobilisations and soft tissue massage), progressive exercise therapy, ice and electrotherapy techniques (including ultrasound, thermal energy and interferential therapy) have a range of therapeutic applications. These include pain relief, reduction of muscle spasm and encouraging tissue healing.

Physiotherapy is identified as an allied health profession (AHP). 'Physiotherapist' and 'physical therapist' are titles protected by law in the UK and the profession is regulated by the Health and Care Professions Council (HCPC); formerly the Health Professions Council (HPC). The HCPC sets mandatory standards of education and training for physiotherapy (HCPC 2012).

In the UK the Chartered Society of Physiotherapy (CSP) offers chartered status to its fully qualified members. The roots of the CSP can be traced to 1894, when four nurses established the Society of Trained Masseuses to give credibility to their profession, which was under threat from individuals offering other services under the guise of massage. The Society gained a Royal Charter in 1920, amalgamated with the Institute of Massage and Remedial Gymnastics and in 1944 adopted its current name. When the National Health Service (NHS) was established in 1948, physiotherapy treatment was prescribed by doctors, dentists or veterinary surgeons. However, in 1977 physiotherapists were granted professional autonomy to assess and treat patients without a referral (Trueland 2008). It is important to recognise that working as an autonomous practitioner does not equate with working independently from other health and social care professionals. This is particularly so within the NHS, where effective team work is emphasised in order to promote high standards of patient care and to avoid potentially disastrous consequences of poor interprofessional working, exemplified by the case of Victoria Climbié (Laming 2003).

Physiotherapists work in a variety of health care settings, including hospitals, general practitioner surgeries and rehabilitation units, as well as in patients' own homes. Physiotherapists working outside the NHS include those who are based in industrial and commercial firms as part of occupational health teams providing services for the workforce. Having a physiotherapist on site reduces the need for staff to travel for outpatient treatment, thereby minimising time lost from work. Physiotherapists also work in private practice, as sports physiotherapists, and in various other working environments. Whilst the NHS has been the traditional employer of physiotherapists in the UK, policy introduced by a Labour Government (DH 2006) and enthusiastically embraced by the subsequent Conservative-Liberal Democrat coalition government, paved the way for new models of service delivery from the third sector. 'Not for profit' organisations such as social enterprises utilise business methods to address social problems (Peckham 2011) and can have a significant role as providers of health care, including physiotherapy.

Governmental plans for developing and supporting the AHPs have identified them as central to the delivery of key priorities of programmes of NHS reforms (DH 2000a, 2000b). Over time, new career pathways, frequently requiring interprofessional collaboration, have developed for physiotherapists, as their skills of assessment, clinical reasoning and treatment have become widely recognised and valued. The development of therapist consultant posts was identified as helping to promote improved quality, service and outcomes for patients, as well as providing new career opportunities, increasing retention of experienced staff and strengthening professional leadership (DH 2000a). Therapist consultants are clinical experts in a particular field, such as a specialist area of physiotherapy practice, and work with senior nursing and medical staff to draw up local care and referral protocols (DH 2000a). The first UK therapist consultant in physiotherapy was appointed in 2002 and CSP records indicated that there were 66 physiotherapy consultants out of approximately 140 AHP consultants in the UK in 2012 (Hunt 2012). The consultant's role focuses on strengthening patient care and services through working across professional boundaries to contribute to strategic planning, service redesign and development, closing the gap between research and clinical practice and developing interprofessional partnerships (Keilty and Bott 2006, Stephenson 2011). In addition to therapist consultants, a growing number of expert physiotherapists' roles involve working beyond the recognised scope of physiotherapy practice. These extended scope practitioners might, for example, spend part of their time working in an outpatient clinic, assessing and diagnosing patients, ordering tests such as X-rays, and referring patients for surgery. Rabey, Morgans and Barrett (2009) highlight that extended scope practitioners are frequently found in UK orthopaedic departments, often managing a patient's entire episode of care, whilst still being accountable to an orthopaedic consultant.

Education

Since 1992 all UK physiotherapy pre-registration courses have been degree programmes and in the early 21st century the threshold for entry onto the HCPC register is a Bachelor degree with honours (HCPC 2012). The length of study varies with the nature of the programme. Many courses last three years, but some higher education institutions offer accelerated programmes, for example, to students already holding an honours degree (or a higher award) in a science-related subject. Part-time programmes enable students to spread their studies over a longer period of time. A number of UK universities offer Master's level pre-registration physiotherapy programmes, which are open to graduates holding a first degree in a relevant subject.

Student physiotherapists need to acquire underpinning theoretical knowledge of, among other things, anatomy, physiology, human movement, biomechanics, pathology, physical principles and electrotherapy. They must develop detailed knowledge of a variety of conditions affecting the cardiovascular, musculoskeletal, neuromuscular and respiratory systems and become adept at employing a range of skills in the examination, assessment and treatment of patients. They are required to learn practical skills such as massage, manual handling techniques, exercise therapy, mobilisation of joints and soft tissues, use of electrotherapy modalities and techniques to improve respiratory function. Other important skills student physiotherapists acquire are those of clinical reasoning and problem solving. As qualified professionals they will be expected to examine and assess patients regularly throughout a programme of treatment and this requires students to become competent in making informed decisions about the most appropriate and effective treatment methods for each individual patient, often in collaboration with other professional groups.

By the time they graduate students will have acquired knowledge, understanding and experience of aspects of professional life that are not specific to physiotherapy. Students develop social skills and understanding of effective interprofessional working and team work as they interact with physiotherapists working in different areas of practice, with a range of other professionals and with members of the public. They work in teams of physiotherapists for specific areas of practice, such as the provision of respiratory care, or the treatment of patients with rheumatological conditions. They also work collaboratively with other health and social care professionals, some of whom may be co-located, and students learn that effective interprofessional working and communication are considered essential for high quality patient care. Undertaking clinical placements in a range of specific areas of patient care, often in different geographical locations, facilitates professional development.

Continuing professional development

After qualification physiotherapists are expected to undertake continuing professional development and they may engage in further training in specialised areas such as ergonomics, sports therapy or veterinary physiotherapy. In 2005, changes to NHS policy enabled physiotherapists, chiropodists/podiatrists and radiographers to train to become supplementary prescribers, a right which to that time had only been available to nurses and pharmacists (DH 2005). An independent prescriber (until 2012 this was a doctor or a dentist) decides in partnership with the supplementary prescriber which patients may benefit from supplementary prescribing and which drugs may be prescribed in this manner as part of a Clinical Management Plan agreed with the patient (DH 2005). In April 2012 changes to the Misuse of Drugs Regulations 2001 gave suitably qualified nurses, midwives and pharmacists independent prescribing rights for many controlled drugs within the scope of their professional expertise, meaning that patients no longer have to wait for a doctor to sign their prescription (DH 2012a). In July 2012, following public consultation, government ministers approved extending independent prescribing rights to advanced practitioner physiotherapists (DH 2012b), representing a major advance in the status of the profession and the potential for transformation of patients' experience of care (Eaton 2012).

Physiotherapists are expected to engage in evidence-based practice, through evaluating and utilising research findings to determine appropriate interventions (HPC 2007). Many physiotherapists are involved in research which may involve collaboration with other professions, not necessarily from health care, in the search for better approaches to patient/client care, health promotion and enhancing physical performance. For example, Clews reported that a key research role for Glenn Hunter, a physiotherapist leading the performance workstream for the UK Sport Research and Innovation Team, was 'to find those minimal but crucial advantages that could propel British athletes towards a bigger haul of medals' (2012: 15) in the 2012 Olympics and beyond, through injury and illness surveillance and redesign of equipment such as rowing boats.

It is not the purpose of this chapter to explain the nature of physiotherapy practice in all health care settings. Rather, a case study will be used to explore the role of the physiotherapist in one specialised area (neurology) in order to highlight profession-specific interventions and to illustrate some aspects of interprofessional working. It should be noted that physiotherapists working in other specialist areas are likely to develop different physiotherapy skills, although effective team working skills are a common feature of professional practice.

CASE STUDY: Bill Grant

Bill Grant is a 55-year-old bus driver born in Jamaica. His wife Marie is also from Jamaica and works full-time in a bank. Bill and Marie have been in the UK for ten years; they have no children and most of their family live overseas. Bill is recovering in hospital after suffering a stroke while gardening, two weeks ago. The stroke was caused by a bleed into the left side of his brain, damaging brain tissue. Each side of the brain controls movement of the opposite side of the body, so the stroke paralysed the right side of Bill's body. When Bill was admitted to the hospital's 20-bedded Specialist Stroke Unit (SSU) from the accident and emergency department he remained unconscious for two days. During this time Bill needed a high level of care from the nursing staff, as well as from the physiotherapists, in order to prevent the potential complications of immobility, including the development of a respiratory infection, debicutus ulcers (pressure sores) or muscle tightness. Two days after his stroke Bill gradually began to regain consciousness. At first he could not move his right arm or leg at all, had weakness in the trunk muscles on his right side and reduced sensation throughout the right side of his body. After a few more days, Bill began to recover some movement in his arm and leg. It became apparent he was having difficulties with speech; he appeared to understand what was said to him but could not respond clearly, jumbling up his sentences. At this stage Bill was not medically ready to go home, even with the care of the Early Supported Discharge team of physiotherapists, occupational therapists, speech and language therapists and specialist nurses.

After two weeks, Bill continues to have difficulty controlling the movement of his right arm and leg and the weakness in his trunk muscles limits the amount of time he can stay upright. The muscles around Bill's shoulder, in his arm and hand remain weak, with marked loss of motor control. He is beginning to regain some movement in the muscles in his right arm and hand, although his hand is still not strong enough to pick up anything, or to be used skilfully during activities such as feeding or dressing.

Bill can now walk short distances with two people helping, one on each side, but finds it difficult to control the muscles in his right leg; he worries that the limb might give way underneath him. In addition to having abnormal motor control of his muscles, Bill is still experiencing some altered sensation, which compounds his movement problems. This seems to be improving slowly, and Bill is undergoing multidisciplinary rehabilitation provided by the stroke specialist team.

Effective multidisciplinary working is the most important aspect of stroke care. Staff should co-ordinate their treatments [and] involve patients and carers in the process...

(RCP 2012: 42).

The provision of coordinated patient care and rehabilitation in the unit is the responsibility of an interprofessional team of occupational therapists, physiotherapists, speech and language therapists, nurses, social workers, a dietician, a clinical psychologist and doctors. The team holds a weekly meeting, chaired by the consultant physician in charge of the unit, to review the progress of each patient and to plan ongoing care. Interprofessional care plans and treatment records for each patient have recently been introduced, which avoids some of the problems associated with keeping separate profession-specific records. This has helped all members of the team remain informed about treatment and care developments, as well as providing insight into the involvement of other professionals. This has fostered effective communication between team members. The unit has 24-hour medical and nursing cover seven days a week, although therapy staff, including physiotherapists, only work during office hours (Monday to Friday 08h30 to 16h30). Patients on the SSU do not normally receive sessions from physiotherapists during the weekend unless they have serious respiratory problems. Should this need arise a patient will be treated by one of the physiotherapists providing weekend cover for the whole hospital. However, the staff are currently considering introducing a seven-day stroke physiotherapy service, a decision based on positive reports in support of the provision of weekend rehabilitation (RCP 2012).

Sasha, one of three physiotherapists working on the SSU, takes the lead in Bill's physiotherapy. However, the physiotherapists work as a team and frequently give each other practical assistance and advice. The physiotherapists are provided with valuable support from an assistant practitioner, who is not a qualified physiotherapist, but who works under their direction, helping patients with exercises, walking practice and so on. The two occupational therapists who work on the SSU have been helping Bill to improve his performance of daily activities such as dressing, feeding and washing. Bill is also receiving help from a speech and language therapist and his speech is improving, although slow progress sometimes makes him frustrated and angry. Post-stroke depression is common (Rashid, Clarke and Rogish 2013) and the SSU team are aware that Bill's communication difficulties could potentially contribute to precipitating this, so a decision has been made for Bill to start regular meetings with the unit's clinical psychologist as a crucial adjunct to the ongoing emotional support that the team offer. The SSU social workers have also introduced themselves to Bill and Marie and regularly attend the SSU team meetings, thereby ensuring that they are fully aware of Bill's progress in preparation for the important part they will play in planning for Bill's discharge home. It is essential that the psychosocial aspects of Bill's care are not neglected, since issues such as untreated mood disturbances following stroke have been linked to higher mortality rates, hospital readmissions, suicide and higher usage of outpatient services (NHS Improvement 2011).

Marie visits Bill each evening after work and comes to see him Saturday and Sunday afternoons. She is looking more tired with each visit. On each occasion Marie checks with the nurses on Bill's progress, although rarely gets to see any of the physiotherapy staff due to the timing of her visits.

Since Bill was first admitted to the SSU, Sasha has assessed him on a regular basis to monitor the recovery of his movement and functional abilities and to decide upon appropriate treatment. Sasha has been working collaboratively with both the nurses and the occupational therapists in encouraging Bill to take particular care of his right arm. Because of Bill's diminished sensation to the right side of his body he is sometimes unaware of his arm being in a potentially damaging position. Sasha has been considering the most appropriate strategies for assisting Bill to become more mobile and to encourage him to regain the use of his affected arm and hand; she has discussed her assessment and proposals with other SSU staff involved in Bill's care and with Bill. They have agreed, for example, that the arrangement of furniture surrounding Bill's bed should encourage him to look across to his right side so as to be more aware of his right arm and hand. Bill's bedside cabinet and table have been placed on the right side of his bed, so that he has to reach over to that side if he wishes to pick something up. Bill is now able to walk to the toilet rather than using a commode, although he is unable to do this if two members of staff are not available to help him. Bill is desperately keen to be able to manage this by himself.

QUESTIONS

- The physiotherapists know that Bill needs to be encouraged at every appropriate opportunity to use his right arm, especially in functional, everyday tasks. Why is this information of relevance to other people?

In answering this question consider not only the members of the health care team on the SSU but also the other people that Bill is likely to encounter.

- Whose role is it to help Bill to walk to the toilet? Justify your answer.
- Bill is getting desperate to manage this task independently; what are the potential consequences of staff regularly being unavailable to help him to the toilet?

Consider both the physical and psychological impact upon Bill, as well as the consequences for Bill's carers.

- Can you think of examples of when the people involved in Bill's care could cause damage to his right shoulder?

When you answer this question try to think as broadly as possible and consider a wide range of activities and situations.

The stability of a shoulder joint relies heavily on normal activity in the surrounding muscles. The partial paralysis of the muscles surrounding Bill's right shoulder joint make it very vulnerable to damage, and everyone involved in his care is aware of how important it is not to traumatise the shoulder whenever they assist Bill. A painful, inflamed shoulder needs to be avoided at all costs.

====== QUESTIONS ======

- What are the potential short-term and long-term problems that could arise from Bill having a painful shoulder?

In answering this question you should consider the consequences for Bill and his carers.

- Who else, in addition to the interprofessional team, needs to be made aware of the potential for causing damage to Bill's shoulder?

You should consider anyone who might come into contact with Bill.

- What advice/support could the team offer Marie at this stage? For example, where should Marie seat herself when she visits Bill?
- What are the potential benefits of a seven-day therapy service?

In answering this question you need to think broadly because the benefits go beyond the impact upon Bill's physical health. For example, consider whether implementing this service has any finanical benefits, and for whom.

Sasha aims to treat Bill twice daily. Treatment sessions last approximately one hour and usually take place in the SSU's rehabilitation gym but are sometimes carried out in the ward, particularly if Sasha has some practical advice or information to share with other team members. Joint treatment sessions, with nurses and occupational therapists for example, give everyone the opportunity to discuss rehabilitation issues and to plan a coordinated approach to patient care.

During treatment Bill is helped to perform functional tasks, specific therapeutic exercises and movement patterns, in order to help him regain movement and function. Two weeks after his stroke Bill's physiotherapy sessions include a variety of activities, designed to tackle his main movement problems. These have been identified in a detailed assessment, carried out over several sessions by Sasha, in consultation with Bill, whose own priority is to walk independently again. He would also like to be able to use his right hand properly, but he is currently more worried about his walking and his inability to speak clearly. The speech and language therapist continues to see Bill regularly and has given him some strategies to help clarify his speech, including encouraging him to speak more slowly than he normally would. Sasha, the occupational therapists and the nurses are aware of this advice and are gently trying to reinforce it in their own sessions.

As Bill is keen to walk, each physiotherapy session includes some activities which work towards this, although specific exercises and functional activities aimed at recovery of more normal movement and function in Bill's arm are also incorporated. Bill is practising walking in parallel bars, with guidance and feedback from Sasha, and is steadily increasing the length of time he can stay on his feet. Bill has been given some exercises to target weakness in specific muscles contributing to his abnormal walking pattern. The physiotherapists are particularly concerned at the marked weakness in the muscles that lift up the foot at the ankle and which prevent the toes from dragging on the floor. A joint therapy session has been arranged between Sasha and one of the occupational therapists, to consider whether Bill might benefit from a splint. Bill is frightened that he is going to trip and fall and a splint might remove this anxiety. The splint can be worn during walking practice, but be removed between walking sessions to enable Bill to build up his muscle strength. Hopefully, in this way, the splint may only be required as a temporary measure, although if the muscle strength does not return, Bill may need to wear a splint to prevent foot drop in the long term. Sasha has some knowledge of splints but recognises the occupational therapist is more skilled in making splints to suit individual patients. The assessment should identify whether Bill requires a tailormade splint or whether he could be supplied with a commercially available splint, in which case a written referral will be made to the hospital's orthotics department.

Bill is making good progress and is starting to ask when he might be able to go home. The team have discussed Bill's discharge at an interprofessional meeting. Although the team feels that Bill is not yet independent enough to go home, they are considering what services Bill might need when he is eventually discharged from the SSU. Sasha thinks it is important that Marie should come along to see what is being done in the physiotherapy sessions and how Bill is progressing. Despite leaving Marie several messages at the SSU reception desk, she has not yet been in touch.

QUESTIONS

- Why might the physiotherapist think that Marie should come to a physiotherapy session?
- What could be preventing Marie from contacting the physiotherapist?
- What are the barriers to effective communication in this case?
- Is there anything that Sasha could consider doing to improve the situation?

The case study provides a small snapshot of some aspects of the physiotherapist's role in Bill's rehabilitation and illustrates how the interprofessional team might interact at various points in Bill's recovery. It demonstrates that while physiotherapists might concentrate on specific activities such as regaining muscle strength, joint range and functional patterns of movement, the holistic management of Bill's rehabilitation is shared between the whole team. Creating formal links with both patients and their carers is considered vital to stroke unit effectiveness (RCP 2012) so it is essential that the team involves Bill and Marie in planning, implementing and evaluating the rehabilitation process.

Decisions regarding Bill's discharge home, and plans for his future care needs, will also be made by the team in conjunction with Bill and Marie. Bill may require ongoing treatment and be referred by Sasha to a physiotherapy outpatient department. Alternatively he may be referred to a community physiotherapist who can see him at home. Bill may also need ongoing input from other professionals, such as the speech and language therapist, and he may require advice from a social worker, for example regarding benefits which he might be entitled to claim. A social worker may also advise Bill on community support groups and help Marie explore her needs as a carer. Marie's needs will have to be carefully considered as she currently has a full-time job. It is very difficult to predict the extent of recovery following a stroke and Bill might be able to return to his job as a bus driver, but only if he regains a high level of functional ability. However, recovery can be slow and many patients who have had a major stroke do not return to full function.

Effective communication systems need to be in place for as long as necessary between members of the interprofessional team, and Bill and Marie, so that Bill's progress can be monitored and any new problems recognised and managed as soon as possible. Hopefully, Bill will continue to recover steadily and his attendance at hospital clinics and his requirement for physiotherapy input will eventually cease. In the long term, Bill and Marie should be given the opportunity to contact a physiotherapist again if they need further help and advice.

Conclusion

This chapter has provided an overview of the physiotherapy profession in the UK. The case study set in a stroke unit has enabled a relatively detailed exploration of a physiotherapist's role in a specialist area of health and social care provision. It has illustrated how being able to work interprofessionally is a critical part of that role and emphasised the importance of engaging the patient and their carers in the decision-making and rehabilitation process.

Where does the uniqueness of being a physiotherapist end and interprofessionalism begin? The question is not a new one. Potts (1996) identified that health professionals will be challenged by having to justify why so many individual groupings, all protective of their professional boundaries, are required for delivery of care and rehabilitation. The NHS Plan articulated clearly that traditional role boundaries are expected to give way to greater flexibility within teams, with staff working under agreed protocols 'that make the best use of all the talents of NHS staff and which are flexible enough to take account of patients' individual needs' (DH 2000b: 83). This is seen as one of the foundations for improving the quality of patient care and providing greater opportunities for staff development.

The physiotherapy profession has come a long way since those four nurses took protection of their profession into their own hands and established the Society of Trained Masseuses. Physiotherapy is set to continue to evolve and in doing so it is not inconceivable that, over time, a new breed of therapist will begin to emerge as a result of the extension of clinical skills and the blurring of professional boundaries.

RECOMMENDED READING

- Catangui E.J. and Slark J. (2012) Development and evaluation of an interdisciplinary training programme for stroke. *British Journal of Neuroscience Nursing* **8**(1): 8–11.
- Royal College of Physicians (2012) *National Clinical Guideline for Stroke Fourth Edition.* www.rcplondon.ac.uk. Accessed June 2013.
- Royal College of Physicians (2012) *Sentinel Stroke National Audit Programme (SSNAP) Acute Organisational Audit Report.* www.rcplondon.ac.uk. Accessed June 2013.
- Reynolds F. (2005) *Communication and Clinical Effectiveness in Rehabilitation.* Edinburgh: Elsevier Butterworth-Heinemann.
- French S. and Sim J. (2004) *Physiotherapy: A Psychosocial Approach.* Edinburgh: Butterworth-Heinemann.

References

Clews G. (2012) Physio aims to give athletes extra edge. *Physiotherapy Frontline* **18**(13): 15.

CSP (Chartered Society of Physiotherapy) (2002) *The Curriculum Framework for Qualifying Programmes in Physiotherapy.* London: CSP.

DH (Department of Health) (2000a) *Meeting the Challenge: A Strategy for the Allied Health Professions.* London: DH.

DH (2000b) *The NHS Plan: A Plan for Investment, a Plan for Reform.* London: DH.

DH (2005) *Supplementary Prescribing by Nurses, Pharmacists, Chiropodists/Podiatrists, Physiotherapists and Radiographers within the NHS in England: A Guide for Implementation.* www.dh.gov.uk. Accessed July 2012.

DH (2006) *Our Health, Our Care, Our Say: A New Direction for Community Services.* www.official-documents.gov.uk. Accessed July 2012.

DH (2012a) *Nurse and Pharmacist Independent Prescribing Changes Announced.* www.dh.gov.uk. Accessed August 2012.

DH (2012b) *Prescribing Powers Proposed for Physiotherapists and Podiatrists.* www.dh.gov.uk. Accessed August 2012.

Eaton L. (2012) Landmark decision gives UK physios a world first in prescribing rights. *Physiotherapy Frontline* **18**(14): 8–9.

HCPC (Health and Care Professions Council) (2012) *Standards of Education and Training.* London: HCPC.

HPC (Health Professions Council) (2007) *Standards of Proficiency – Physiotherapists.* www.hcpc-uk.org. Accessed July 2012.

Hunt L. (2012) Members are being asked to provide information on allied health professional (AHP) consultant posts in their area to ensure the UK database is up to date. *Physiotherapy Frontline* **18**(5). www.csp.org.uk. Accessed June 2012.

Keilty S.E.J. and Bott J. (2006) Opportunities in acute and chronic respiratory physiotherapy: recent developments in the UK. *Physical Therapy Reviews* **11**: 44–8.

Laming, Lord (2003) *The Victoria Climbié Inquiry: Report of an Inquiry by Lord Laming.* Norwich: HMSO.

NHS Improvement (2011) *Psychological Care after Stroke: Improving Stroke Services for People with Cognitive and Mood Disorders.* www.improvement.nhs.uk. Accessed June 2013.

Peckham S. (2011) Social enterprise pathfinders. *The Lancet UK Policy Matters.* http://ukpolicy-matters.thelancet.com. Accessed July 2012.

Potts J. (1996) Physiotherapy in the next century: opportunities and challenges. *Physiotherapy* **82**: 150–5.

Rabey M., Morgans S. and Barrett C. (2009) Orthopaedic physiotherapy practitioners: surgical and radiological referral rates. *Clinical Governance: An International Journal* **14**(1): 15–19.

Rashid N., Clarke C. and Rogish M. (2013) Post-stroke depression and expressed emotion. *Brain Injury* **27**(2): 223–38.

RCP (Royal College of Physicians) (2012) *Sentinel Stroke National Audit Programme (SSNAP) Acute Organisational Audit Report.* www.rcplondon.ac.uk. Accessed June 2013.

Stephenson K. (2011) Professional development: integrating the consultant physiotherapist role within a musculoskeletal interface service. *Musculoskeletal Care* **9**: 49–53.

Trueland J. (2008) Diamond service. *Physiotherapy Frontline* **14**(12). www.csp.org.uk. Accessed July 2012.

CHAPTER 11

Police

Peter Kennison and Robin Fletcher

Introduction

This chapter offers an outline of the nature and scope of policing by examining its role and working relationships with other agencies. In particular, we discuss the interprofessional relationships that developed between the police, social services and health services in England and Wales and examine how these partnerships can fail. The failures to protect both Victoria Climbié and Peter Connelly (Baby P), utilised as case studies in this chapter, were rightly condemned by public and the media when evidence implicated poor communication and ineffective cooperation between partner agencies as major contributing factors. When the police fail to act in accordance with public and media expectations, they are rightly called to account. These expectations raise at least three questions: what exactly is the role of the police; can, or more importantly, should the police be 'placid' partners when dealing with violent domestic crimes; and do the police possess the skills necessary to achieve satisfactory conclusions in these types of criminal investigations? We review how the role has become fragmented, interchangeable, and complex such that the police are no longer entirely sure about what they are expected to deliver.

The role of police

In 1829, then Home Secretary and founder of modern policing, Sir Robert Peel, set out first principles stating: 'It should be understood at the outset that the principal objective to be attained is the prevention of crime' (cited in

140

Alderson 1979: 198). To achieve this, uniformed officers would patrol streets (Critchley 1967, Emsley 1996) deterring potential offenders by their mere presence (Reiner 1992). Success of these patrols depended on local knowledge, trust between officers and citizens, and informal control mechanisms. Initially effective in non-migratory communities with low public expectations, the role of the police officer was perceived as peace keeper and mediator, with occasional law enforcement using 'common sense', intuition and fellow officer support. The more recent idea of an 'omni-competent' constable reflects police as instantly contactable, and capable of dealing with any problem (Bittner 1991). As Morgan and Newburn summarise:

> The police frequently are the only 24-hour service agency available to respond to those in need. The result is that the police handle everything from unexpected child births, skid row alcoholics, drug addicts, emergency psychiatric cases, family fights, landlord-tenant disputes, and traffic violations, to occasional incidents of crime.
>
> (1997: 79).

High visibility policing continued until the advent of requirements for efficiency and effectiveness. The post-World War II welfare state of a National Health Service, state-owned housing provision, improved education, and well-paid employment raised expectations of state provision, intervention and control (Christie 1977). Migration to New Towns with concomitant collapsing of informal social control mechanisms (Wilson and Kelling 1982) resulted in more calls for police intervention.

The 1962 Royal Commission (Cmd 1,728 1962) introduced a policing model that moved officers from streets into vehicles to facilitate rapid police responses to calls for assistance (Emsley 1996, Home Office 1967). This 'fire brigade' policing (McLaughlin and Muncie 1996) with its seemingly 'machismo' approach often dealt quickly with incidents but at the expense of community cohesion and a failure to appreciate the need for long-term solutions.

The preventative activity of the few remaining foot patrols tried to retain the confidence of local communities and develop the information flows necessary for developing crime intelligence. This policing activity re-emerged in the aftermath of the inner-city riots of the 1980s in the attempt to re-establish trust and cooperation between police and the community. Despite evidence that foot patrols are ineffective (Kelling, Pate, Dieckman and Brown 1974, Morgan and Newburn 1997), community policing continues, supported by an 'extended police family', of Police Community Safety Officers, Neighbourhood Wardens, and private uniformed security staff supplementing 'warranted' police officers. This 'neighbourhood' policing model seeks to 'address the gap between the public perception of rising crime and the falling crime rate' (Tuffin, Morris and Poole 2006: x) and appears to be an exercise in public relations.

Social and political context

Following a period of relative political, social and economic calm, the late 1970s and early 1980s saw an increase in public disorder, notably:

a. industrial disputes;
b. demonstrations and counter-demonstrations;
c. recreational meetings, e.g. football matches and the bank holiday clashes between mods and skinheads;
d. spontaneous attacks on police in inner-city areas. (O'Byrne1981: 15)

The first three suggest political and social instability; the fourth indicates loss of respect for a police force accused of racism, sexism and heavy-handedness (Hall, Critcher, Jefferson *et al.* 1978, Lea and Young 1993, Solomos 1993) signalling a low point in police community cooperation. The 1978 election of Margaret Thatcher heralded a politicisation of policing (Downes and Morgan 1994) as the left sought to direct activities at social injustice and community safety through local unelected bodies (Fletcher and Stenson 2009), while the right sought to break trade union power and use central control to impose law and order on all.

In response to rising street crime in Brixton in the early 1980s, operation 'Swamp 81' (Brake and Hale 1992, CRE 1981, Scarman 1981) saw large numbers of police officers stop and search nearly 1,000 predominantly black youths in a four-day period (McLaughlin and Muncie 1996). Sparking the inner-city riots of the 1980s and changing the nature of policing, the militaristic police response to the riots and in battles with the trade unions were condemned by the left as an attack on civil rights but supported by the right as the legitimate use of force for law enforcement purposes.

Developing partnerships

This social conflict changed the direction of the Thatcher government from law enforcement towards community prevention tackling issues of causation (Crawford 1998). The Five Towns Initiative, Safer Cities, Housing Action Trusts, and the Single Regeneration Bids are examples of partnership projects that challenged the concept of the police as the sole crime control and prevention management agency. Government Circular 8/84 identified crime prevention as a whole community task (Home Office 1984) recognising that the police alone could not tackle crime. Partnerships emerged ad hoc as different agencies and some sections of the community began working together. An early partnership, the police/community consultation groups, imposed by the Police and Criminal Evidence Act 1984 (www.legislation.gov.uk) in response to Lord Scarman's (1981) report into the inner city riots, was followed by a flurry of partnerships reviewed by the Morgan Report (Home Office 1991) whose recommendations were rejected by the Thatcher government.

What are partnerships?

Within months of election, the 1997 New Labour government introduced the Crime and Disorder Act 1998 (www.legislation.gov.uk) as the major thrust of its crime reduction programme (Home Office 1998) using the previously discarded Morgan Report as a blueprint. Intended to make the police and local authorities jointly accountable for reductions in crime and anti-social behaviour, it had two key elements: extensive public consultation; and statutorily bringing together the local authority Chief Executive and the local senior Police Officer as a 'Responsible Authority'. This Responsible Authority included other statutory and voluntary agencies, victim support services, the business sector, and community groups in developing holistic solutions. Some of the more innovative partnerships to emerge include: Crime and Disorder Reduction Partnerships; Child Protection Teams; Youth Offender Teams; and Multi Agency Public Protection Arrangements.

Specialist skills

The focus on community engagement was an attempt to deliver on Peel's primary objective but may have overshadowed a second objective set out by the first Metropolitan Police Commissioner, Sir Richard Mayne, in 1829 as 'the next [object is] that of detection and punishment of offenders if crime is committed' (Metropolitan Police 2012).

The case of Stephen Lawrence highlighted gaps in investigative practice and showed that identifying a suspect and proving a case beyond reasonable doubt is complex and difficult. A lack of investigative training can be traced to late 1970s and early 1980s research (Bottomley and Coleman 1981, Burrows and Tarling 1987) suggesting most crime is solved by the public and indicating little need for police skills beyond those of the ordinary constable. Over the intervening years this approach failed to take into account 'Changes to the legal framework of criminal investigations' and 'Technological and procedural changes to the investigative process' (Stelfox 2009: 33) that added complexity to investigative processes.

In addition to managing crime scenes, gathering evidence, identifying witnesses, tracing suspects and so on, senior investigating officers are expected to complete strategy and policy documents to justify decision making; manage an intrusive media; deal with public expectations; provide family liaison officers for the more traumatic incidents; work closely with other agencies; and be sensitive to those 'signal' crimes (Innes 2005) with wider community impact. To address this shortfall of skills a Professionalising Investigation Programme was introduced in 2005 'to drive through new standards of investigation at all levels' (NCPE 2005: 1) and when coupled with the 'new methods and procedures' in police child protection pro-activity, promoted a safer environment for all. It is of concern therefore to read that 'Even with all the systems implemented and prevention strategies in place, it is an unfortunate fact that some children will still be abused and killed by their carers' (Bourlet 2008: 126).

Youth Offending Teams bring police, social workers, education workers, youth workers, and probation officers together to deal with crime committed by young people. Such partnership working presupposes participating agencies will function effectively. The following two cases illustrate failures in child protection partnership working, even when lessons should have been learned and when new procedures should have provided protection for the child. The inquiry into the death of Victoria Climbié highlighted problems arising from ineffective working relationships between the police, health and social services. Some of the difficulties are identified below.

CASE STUDY: Victoria Climbié

Victoria Climbié, a black child born in the Ivory Coast, was entrusted into the care of Marie-Theresa Kouao, an aunt, by her parents who wanted a better life for her in England. She arrived in the UK on 24th April 1999 with her identity subverted to that of Kouao's daughter. Travelling as EU citizens they went to accommodation in Acton and then Harlesden. During later visits to Ealing Social Services the staff noticed Victoria was dressed less well than her 'mother' (Laming 2003).

Within two months, injuries on Victoria had been noticed. Kouao explained away scars as resulting from an escalator fall. Three days after Kouao met Carl Manning, a friend of Kouoa was sufficiently concerned about Victoria to telephone Brent Social Services twice. By the end of this tragic affair, there had been contact with Haringey Social Services, Enfield Social Services and the Tottenham Child and Family Centre (Laming 2003): all to no avail. Not one of the agencies empowered to protect children emerge from this Inquiry with much credit (Laming 2003: 3).

Child Protection Teams

Comprising police officers, social workers and other professionals, Child Protection Teams were established to focus on protecting the interests of child victims rather than prosecution and conviction (Fido and Skinner 1999).

CASE STUDY continued

Victoria was first seen for injuries later described as non-accidental (Laming 2003) at the Central Middlesex Hospital on 14th July 1999. The paediatric registrar recorded numerous injuries on Victoria's body and Brent Social Services were informed of her admission for observation and further examination. The next day another doctor diagnosed scabies as causing Victoria's injuries and she left hospital. One week later, and concerned about facial scalding, Kouao took Victoria to the North Middlesex Hospital. Victoria spent 13 nights in the paediatric ward. On her third visit to hospital on 25th February 2000 Victoria was declared dead aged eight years and three months.

Laming noted the case was initially given low priority despite evidence suggesting serious physical injury. The victim was in hospital and with social services agreement was placed under police protection. The officer went off duty and failed to visit Victoria, a factor which Laming suggested was a crucial error of judgement (Laming 2003: 299). By the time of her death Victoria had been brought to the attention of five social service agencies (two in the same borough) and had three visits to two separate hospitals. Whilst treatment rightly takes priority, many professional partners working in child protection often see crime as solely a matter for the police. This does not reflect a culture of partnership.

▨ What are your responsibilities in reporting to the police suspected cases of deliberate harm to a child?

Confusion of roles and responsibilities

The Laming Report illustrates serious failings of the police. In cases of suspected harm to a child the police are the lead investigative agency responsible for making enquiries, collecting information, and evaluating evidence for criminal prosecutions. They submit case files to the Crown Prosecution Service where, if sufficient evidence exists, prosecution will be pursued. In Victoria's case roles and responsibilities were blurred (Laming 2003: 324) and although child protection is a primary function of social services, Laming pointed out that the police should have conducted a parallel investigation into the crime reported against her (Laming 2003: 306); Laming also noted that the child protection officers had been unsure regarding their exact role and responsibilities within the context of Child Protection Teams, especially regarding not being the lead agency (Laming 2003: 306). Had this uncertainty been discussed within the team a clearer understanding of the roles and responsibilities of different professionals might have facilitated more effective interprofessional working.

▨ What factors might result in confusion regarding the roles and responsibilities of different professional groups?
▨ What factors might inhibit a junior member of one profession questioning the views of a senior member of another profession?

Laming highlighted deficiencies in both supervision and training. Had junior officers been effectively supervised mistakes might have been avoided (Laming 2003: 303). Laming recommended all child protection officers receive training in challenging the views of others (Laming 2003: 321). Interprofessional education (CAIPE 1997) would appear suitable to facilitate the development of the knowledge, skills and attitudes required to work in interprofessional child protection teams.

Group behaviour – the problems of (organisational) culture

While individual failures are important, group behaviour also plays a part and depends on group norms, beliefs, understandings and shared goals. Organisational goals are set by established hierarchies and internal conflict can arise when organisational and group goals differ. The group dynamics of cultural structures or vertical hierarchies reflect the differences in cultural groups. Cultural differences in Crime and Disorder Partnerships were highlighted in a report (Home Office 1991) where particular attention was drawn to 'Local Authority', 'police centred', and 'police headquarters' models. Crawford (1998) notes that differences in coordination, structure and resourcing within each model reflects agency role, processes and organisation. Vertical hierarchies separate lines of communication, supervision and management functions within individual agencies. Police frustration often manifests as good humoured banter used to diffuse tense situations that otherwise might deteriorate into confrontation. Rooted in police culture, this reaction is a by-product of performance occupational (and therefore, blame) culture as a way of coping with competing local, national and organisational demands (Kennison 2008).

During the Laming inquiry police representatives provided many examples of good working relationships with social services. However, some within the police reported feeling some social services professionals held unhelpful stereotypical views of the police as heavy-handed (Laming 2003: 312) and focused on securing convictions rather than on the interests of the child (Laming 2003: 312); others perceived social service staff as inflexible and unprepared to negotiate mutually convenient times and places for strategy meetings (Laming 2003: 312). In this environment trust and cooperation broke down to the detriment of the child. Laming noted a sense of inequality between the agencies and he criticised the police for failing to challenge this. According to Laming, child protection strategy meetings should reflect shared multiagency responsibility (Laming 2003: 321).

QUESTIONS

- What stereotypical views might be held regarding the police?
- What stereotypes might be held of other professional groups with whom you might be required to work?

Mutual respect, a critical attribute of collaborative working (Stapleton1998), is facilitated through open and honest communication enabling professionals to develop understanding of each other's perspectives. Had the perceptions of inequality, inflexibility, and stereotyping been openly discussed this may have provided a platform for mutual understanding, flexible patterns of working, and a more equal distribution of power.

CASE STUDY continued

On 12th January 2001 Marie-Theresa Kouao and Carl Manning were convicted and jailed for life, for the murder of Victoria (Anna) Climbié. The post mortem showed she died from hypothermia resulting from malnourishment, a damp environment and restricted movement (Laming 2003). She had 128 separate injuries showing that she had been beaten with a range of both sharp and blunt instruments. The last days of her short life were spent living in a cold unheated bathroom, bound hand and foot inside a bin bag lying in her own urine and excrement. To some involved this had been the worst case of child abuse they had ever seen.

There were at least 12 key occasions when the relevant services had an opportunity to intervene (Laming 2003). These warning signs occurred when Victoria had been taken or been referred to hospital emergency departments, social services departments or the police. As a result Victoria was left to die abandoned, unheard, in agony and alone. Laming suggests this represented gross and inexcusable failure.

CASE STUDY: Peter Connelly (Baby P)

On 3rd August 2007, Peter Connelly, aged 17 months, was found dead in his cot 48 hours after a doctor failed to identify his severe injuries, including a broken spine. He was on Haringey Council's child protection register throughout eight months of abuse in which he suffered more than 50 injuries. His family were seen 60 times by agencies, including local authority social workers. Peter was the subject of extensive inquiries by the child protection review panel comprising all agencies with an interest in his welfare. Unlike the Victoria Climbié case, there was a properly constituted panel to protect Peter Connelly.

Haringey Social Services had been the focus of the national outcry over Victoria Climbié. Had anything been learned?

Peter's stepfather, Steven Barker and his brother, Jason Owen, were convicted of causing or allowing the child's death, a charge to which Peter's mother, Tracey Connelly, had previously pleaded guilty. The case was complex (Garboden 2010) with similar errors to those seen in the case of Victoria Climbié but with a different pattern of partnership working. Haringey Social Services once more bore the brunt of criticism with two social workers admitting misconduct at a later inquiry. This said, the police and the health service also made errors of judgement.

Disagreement and conflict

Like the Victoria Climbié case there was disagreement, conflict and blame between agencies with publically aired recriminations following intense media interest. Sharon Shoesmith (head of Haringey's Social Services) was publically sacked by Ed Balls (Home Secretary); a situation which she challenged and it was found that due process had not been used, she had been scapegoated and that her dismissal was unlawful (Butler 2011). Documents seen by *The Guardian* relating to the original full serious case review show police officers made a series of mistakes missing the chance to charge Baby P's mother with assault several weeks before his death (Ramesh and Butler 2010). The officers could have visited the home with social services and should have kept detailed notes. A specialist identified to undertake an independent medical review requested by the Crown Prosecution Service did not complete the review because the detective in charge was transferred to another section in the Metropolitan police without formally handing over the case: a clear breach of standard operating procedures. For two months the case just drifted (Ramesh and Butler 2010).

CASE STUDY continued

Peter Connelly was first taken to the Whittington hospital with extensive bruising in December 2006. Doctors thought his injuries suspicious and he was put on Haringey Council's child protection register. Failures in investigative procedures mirror those of the Victoria Climbié case with grave errors of duty failing Peter Connelly – his bruises remained unphotographed for one week; his home (a potential crime scene) was not photographed; and evidence was not preserved and lost (Butler 2011). Once again fundamental crime investigation errors were made.

As with the Victoria Climbié case, partnership working in the supervision of Peter Connelly, produced a conflict of opinion in situations where ideologies, traditions and interests diverge that shows each group possesses different levels of authority, power and control. Variations in specialist knowledge and expertise and in access to human and material resources abound (Crawford 1998). Budgetary constraints may discourage social workers from taking legal safeguards such as Care Orders or Emergency Protection Orders (Davies 2009). So even when evidence is submitted for a case review meeting consideration (as Laming requires), if no further action is taken to safeguard the child the police become frustrated and disinterested. In this case the police concentrated on investigation rather than prevention (Davies 2008). Some specialist police knowledge will conflict with other partners especially in terms of investigation, as not all social workers have access to joint investigation training courses. Some agencies have superior legal authority – for example, unlike social services the police have legal authority to access premises by force if access is denied. This dominance frequently attracts criticism and resistance from other partners (Kennison 2008).

But what if there is conflict and difference of opinion between the police and other members relating to further action in protecting children? The police raised concerns with the partnership panel only days before Peter Connelly's death. The serious case review stated:

> that not only were team managers wrong (given Baby P's past injuries) not to undertake care proceedings but also that whilst the police were correct in raising concerns over the child's welfare, the way they intervened was wrong.
>
> (LSCB 2009)

Munro (2010) puts this type of error down to a lack of training and understanding on the part of police, social workers and managers.

In identifying significant weakness, the findings of the Joint Area Review showed arrangements for the leadership and management of safeguarding by local authority and partner agencies in Haringey were inadequate (LSCB 2009: 5). The failure of the Local Safeguarding Children Board to provide sufficient challenge to member agencies was compounded by the lack of an independent chairperson. There was inadequate communication and collaboration between social care, health services and police in assessment, planning and review of cases of vulnerable children and young people. This often resulted in a failure in all agencies to identify or address the needs of those at immediate risk of harm. The quality of front-line practice across agencies was inconsistent and ineffectively monitored. Child protection plans were found to be 'generally poor'; arrangements for scrutinising performance across council partnerships were insufficiently developed and failed to provide systematic support or appropriate challenges to managers and practitioners. In all agencies, standards of record keeping were inconsistent and often poor. There was over-reliance on quantitative data to measure social care, health and police performance, without sufficiently robust analysis of the underlying quality of service provision and practice (LSCB 2009).

Conclusion

Police accountability is complicated and diffuse. The role of police has shifted from prevention to law enforcement to actuarial justice. Within this latter role prominence was paid first to the maintenance of public order and then to a return of community-based policing methods responding to the needs of the community whilst working in partnership with other agencies to solve common problems.

In the case of Victoria Climbié, the prosecution rested with the police yet they perceived this as a decision for social services as the lead agency. In both cases there were differences of opinion regarding the role of police not only by the police themselves but also by social workers. This confusion hindered investigation, training and collaboration. Both cases illustrate that individuals from different agencies working separately with little consultation leads to inadequate cross-agency communication and problem solving.

Originally an impressive model of good partnership practice, the Child Protection Team and lately Child Abuse Investigation Teams investigations in both cases failed because of inadequate investigative skills, insufficient experience and poor training. Blurred individual and partnership roles, disjointed lines of accountability as well as ineffective internal communication, supervision and management further compounded the problem. If partnerships are to function effectively, accurate information sharing is key to reliable problem solving and decision making.

RECOMMENDED READING

- Beckett C. (2007) *Child Protection – An Introduction*. Sage: London.
- Kennison P. and Goodman A. (eds) (2008) *Children as Victims*. Exeter: Learning Matters.
- Watkin A., Lindqvist S., Black J. and Watts F. (2009) Report on the implementation and evaluation of an interprofessional learning programme for inter-agency child protection teams. *Child Abuse Review* 18(3): 151–67.
- For a general introduction to roles within policing see: *www.policerecruitment.homeoffice.gov.uk*.

References

Alderson J. (1979) *Policing Freedom*. Plymouth: Latimer Trend.

Bittner E. (1991) The functions of the police in modern society. In Klockars C.B. and Mastrofski S.D. (eds) *Thinking about Police*. New York: McGraw-Hill, pp. 35–51.

Bottomley K. and Coleman C. (1981) *Understanding Crime Rates*. Farnborough: Gower.

Bourlet C. (2008) Minimising the risk to children and young people: the police response. In Kennison P. and Goodman A. (eds) *Children as Victims*. Exeter: Learning Matters, pp. 115–27.

Brake M. and Hale C. (1992) *Public Order and Private Lives*. London: Routledge.

Burrows J. and Tarling R. (1987) The investigation of crime in England and Wales. *British Journal of Criminology* 27: 229–51.

Butler P. (2011) 'Child protection work facing recruitment crisis after Baby P tragedy' *The Guardian* Friday 27th May 2011. www.guardian.co.uk. Accessed October 2013.

CAIPE (Centre for the Advancement of Interprofessional Education) (1997) *Interprofessional Education – A Definition*. London: CAIPE Bulletin **13.**

Christie N. (1977) Conflicts as property. *British Journal of Criminology* 17: 1–15.

Cmd 1,728 (1962) *The Final Report on the Royal Commission on the Police*. London: HMSO.

Crawford A. (1998) *Crime Prevention and Community Safety*. London: Longman.

CRE (Commission for Racial Equality) (1981) *CRE's Submission under Part II of Lord Scarman's Enquiry into the Brixton Disorders*. London: CRE.

Critchley T.A. (1967) *A History of Police in England and Wales*. London: Constable.

Davies L. (2008) Reforms have been imposed at the expense of protecting children. *The Guardian*. Joepublicblog posted 12th December.

Davies L. (2009) Submission to the Progress Review of Lord Laming: www.lizdavies.net/cpa/. Accessed March 2012.

Downes D. and Morgan R. (1994) Hostages to fortune? The politics of law and order in postwar Britain. In Maguire M., Morgan R. and Reiner R. (eds), *The Handbook of Criminology*. Oxford: Oxford Press.

Emsley C. (1996) The history of crime and crime control institutions c1770–c1945. In Maguire M. Morgan R., and Reiner R. (eds), *The Oxford Handbook of Criminology*. Oxford: Clarendon, pp. 149–82.

Fido M. and Skinner K. (1999) *The Official Encyclopaedia of Scotland Yard*. London: Virgin Press.

Fletcher R. and Stenson K. (2009) Governance and the London Metropolitan Police Service *Policing, A Journal of Policy and Practice* 3: 12–21.

Garboden M. (2010) Baby Peter case in Haringey. www.communitycare.co.uk. Accessed February 2012.

Hall S., Critcher C., Jefferson T., Clarke J. and Roberts B. (1978) *Policing the Crisis: Mugging the State and Law and Order*. London: Macmillan.

Home Office (1967) *Police Manpower, Equipment and Efficiency*. London: HMSO.

Home Office, Department of Education and Science, Department of the Environment, Department of Health and Social Security and Welsh Office (1984) *Crime Prevention* (Home Office Circular 8/1984). London: Home Office.

Home Office (1991) *Safer Communities: The Local Delivery of Crime Prevention through the Partnership Approach* (the Morgan Report). London: Home Office.

Home Office (1998) *Crime and Disorder Act Guidelines*. London: HMSO.

Innes M. (2005) What's your problem: signal crimes and citizen-focused problem-solving (Reaction Essay). *Criminology and Public Policy* 4(2): 187–200.

Kelling G., Pate T., Dieckman D. and Brown C. (1974) *The Kansas City Preventive Patrol Experiment: A Summary Report*. Washington DC: Police Foundation.

Kennison P. (2008) Learning from mistakes: understanding police failure. In Kennison P. and Goodman A. (eds), *Children as Victims*. Exeter: Learning Matters.

Laming Lord (2003) *Inquiry into the Death of Victoria Climbié*. London: The Stationery Office.

Lea J. and Young J. (1993) *What Is to Be Done about Law and Order*. London: Pluto.

LSCB (Local Safeguarding Children Board) (2009) Serious Case Review – baby Peter. www.haringeylscb.org. Accessed November 2012.

McLaughlin E. and Muncie J. (1996) *Controlling Crime*. London: Sage.

Metropolitan Police (2012) History of the Metropolitan Police. www.met.police.uk. Accessed November 2012.

Morgan R. and Newburn T. (1997) *The Future of Policing*. Oxford: Clarendon Press.

Munro E. (2010) The Munro review of Child Protection. www.education.gov.uk. Accessed November 2012.

NCPE (National Centre for Policing Excellance) (2005) *Codes of Practice*. Bramshill: Centrex.

O'Byrne M. (1981) The role of the police. In Pope D.W. and Weiner N.L. (eds), *Modern Policing*. London: Croom Helm, pp. 11–21.

Ramesh R. and Butler P. (2010) Baby P files show police left him in danger – Lawyers say. *The Guardian* Friday 2nd April 2010. www.guardian.co.uk. Accessed October 2013.

Reiner R. (1992) *The Politics of Police*. London: Harvester Wheatsheaf.

Scarman Lord (1981) *The Brixton Disorders 10–12 April 1981: Report of an Inquiry by the Rt. Hon. The Lord Scarman O.B.E.* London: HMSO.

Solomos J. (1993) *Race and Racism in Britain*. London: Macmillan.

Stapleton S.R. (1998) Team-building: making collaborative practice work. *Journal of Nurse-Midwifery* **43**: 12–18.

Stelfox P. (2009) *Criminal Investigation: An Introduction to Principles and Practice*. Collumpton: Willan.

Tuffin R., Morris J. and Poole A. (2006) *An Evaluation of the Impact of the National Reassurance Policing Programme*. Home Office Research. Study 296. London: Home Office.

Wilson J. and Kelling G. (1982) Broken windows. *The Atlantic Monthly* March.

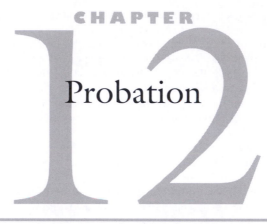

CHAPTER 12

Probation

Jane Lindsay and Kuljit Sandhu

Introduction

Probation has its origins in the 19th century with the provision of voluntary support to offenders appearing before police courts. The Probation of Offenders Act 1907 (www.probation.ie) created the probation service and the appointment of probation officers, with a clear mission to 'advise, support and befriend' offenders under supervision (GB 1907, Ch 17: 5). Since then, like other public services, probation's role and purpose has been transformed and professionalised. Its current form was established by the Criminal Justice and Court Services Act 2000 (www.legislation.gov.uk) in April 2001. Probation's statutory aims are currently to reduce reoffending, protect the public and ensure that offenders are aware of the effects of crime on victims. Probation makes an important contribution to community safety and crime reduction. Probation works jointly with statutory, private sector and voluntary, community and social enterprise service providers including police, prison, health, victim support, social services and housing to manage and rehabilitate offenders effectively in custody and in the community.

This chapter outlines probation's approach to working with other professionals, offenders, victims and communities. An outline of the organisational structure of the service both nationally and locally is provided and some key policy trends which may influence interprofessional work are highlighted. Some of the issues about probation values are discussed. Information is provided about staff and training and key probation tasks focusing on work with other professionals. The chapter concludes with an overview of some of the challenges of and vision for working interprofessionally to promote justice and rehabilitation.

National organisational structure

Like many public services, probation has been subject to many changes in its organisational structure. In May 2013, the government announced the creation of a new public sector national English probation service which will commence from autumn 2014 with public sector probation having 'a distinct identity for Wales, facilitating links and relationships with the Welsh Government' (GB 2013: 25). This new strategy (GB 2013) outlines new governmental arrangements for reform of the provision of rehabilitation services. From 2014, the public sector probation service will be responsible for pre-sentence advice to court, assessing the risk an offender poses to the public, and directly managing those subject to Multi Agency Public Protection Arrangements and those who pose the highest risk to the public. The provision of services to offenders who are not deemed to constitute such a high risk to the public will be opened up to private sector providers who will sub-contract with Voluntary, Community and Social Enterprise (VCSE) providers to provide services. Private and VCSE providers will be paid by a combined payment mechanism of a fee for the service and payment by results; results meaning 'an agreed reduction in the number of offenders who go on to commit further offences, and a reduction in the number of further offences committed by the cohort of offenders for which they are responsible' (GB 2013: 5). Having a diverse market for rehabilitation services is expected to lead to increased opportunities for other agencies to contribute directly to working to rehabilitate offenders in the community and more interprofessional work.

The work of probation is scrutinised by the National Offender Management Service (NOMS) within the Ministry of Justice. NOMS deals with probation, prisons and the private and the VCSE sector providers to manage offenders in the community and prison to ensure that they are punished, and that their reoffending is reduced. Since 2007, the concept of *end-to-end offender management* (Offender Management Act 2007 – www.legislation.gov.uk) has guided practice. This means that the progress offenders make in prison should be built on in the community. One of the objectives of NOMS is to ensure value for money and effectiveness in reducing reoffending.

Probation is a Responsible Authority on the Crime and Disorder Reduction Partnerships set up to develop community safety strategies by working together to protect the public (Crime and Disorder Act 1998, s. 5 and s. 6 – www. legislation.gov.uk). Members of these partnerships include the police, local authorities and a range of representatives from local community services, for example, education, social services, youth services, neighbourhood watch, victim support and local employers. Partnerships are required to conduct and publish an audit of local crime and disorder problems, determine priorities for action, devise and publish a strategy, and monitor and review progress.

Public perceptions of probation

Public recognition of probation and rehabilitation services seems poor. The British Crime Survey (Jansson 2008) found that only 20 per cent of the public considered that probation was either doing a good or an excellent job. The government has recognised that there is a need to take measures to improve public confidence in community penalties. One example is the Casey report (2008) which proposed that people sentenced to undertake unpaid work – community payback (formerly community service) – wear distinctive fluorescent tabards which identify them as offenders. There is no research as yet as to whether the measure has improved public perceptions of probation and it has been criticised as an emotive response which misinterprets public perceptions of punishment and rehabilitation (Maruna and King 2008). A more positive response is suggested by Allen and Hough (2007) of encouraging greater engagement of the public and communities in working with people sentenced to community sentences on the grounds that 'increasing involvement can impact forcefully on attitudes and might therefore be a way of producing more positive opinions' (Allen and Hough 2007: 584). The new arrangements for rehabilitation services, with greater involvement of the VCSE sector may produce this engagement and create more opportunities for interprofessional work and lead to better opportunities for working collaboratively with individuals and families.

Probation values

Until the final decade of the 20th century probation values were rooted firmly in the values of social work. Changing policy agendas which emphasised punishment and control together with changes from social work to probation-specific qualifications led to probation 'floundering in attempts to establish clearly identifiable values which might be perceived as legitimate by government, practitioners and the public alike' (Gelsthorpe 2007: 490). The value statements issued by governmental bodies charged with national leadership of probation (for example, NOMS 2011) have been criticised as being an operational methodology which fails to think about values coherently (Gelsthorpe 2007).

There has been considerable debate about what should constitute professional values in probation. Nellis (2002) argues for community justice values, and that all in the community should be involved in the pursuit of ensuring community safety, restorative justice and reducing the excessive use of imprisonment. Weaver and McNeill (2007) point to the need to promote redemption and to recognise, encourage and confirm the efforts made by offenders to change and to desist from criminal activity. There is increasing interest in promoting positive ethics of probation around the discourse of human rights as this encompasses the rights of victims and the rights and responsibilities of offenders, while recognising that lawful limitations on offenders' rights are a necessary consequence of punishment (Gelsthorpe 2007). Canton (2011) highlights the need for probation to explain its work openly to the public, provide evidence-led opportunities for rehabilitation and promote the importance of working in partnership with other agencies.

Staff and training

Probation staff includes a number of different professional groups, including probation officers, probation service officers and psychologists. *Probation officers* are responsible for report writing for the courts and the Parole Board as well as undertaking risk assessment and management jointly with police and prison service to manage the most dangerous offenders. They also deliver specialist rehabilitative programmes. *Probation service officers,* who are not qualified probation officers, undertake tasks such as court work and working as hostel officers. Some staff members are seconded to work in Youth Offending Teams (YOTs), prisons and other public protection and crime prevention or reduction partnership agencies. (For more information about YOTs see www.justice.gov.uk).

Before 1997 a probation officer was required to be a qualified social worker. Then probation developed its own specialist Diploma in Probation Studies with a specific focus on enforcement, rehabilitation and public protection. A national probation qualifying framework to replace the diploma was developed in 2010 that combines academic study with work-based learning. Private and VCSE sectors providing rehabilitation services are expected to provide a workforce with appropriate levels of training. They may access the Probation Qualifications Framework or other professional or vocational qualifications.

An overview of key probation roles and tasks

Probation works primarily with people aged 18 and over who have been convicted of offences. Services provided include pre-sentence advice to court, assessing the risk an offender poses to the public, managing those subject to Multi Agency Public Protection Arrangements and supervising those who pose the highest risk to the public, including those released from prison. Probation also advises the parole board on release decisions; provides a victim liaison service in cases where offenders are sentenced to 12 months or over for violent or sexual offences; manages approved premises (hostels) and takes action when people have breached the conditions of sentences and licences.

Since the introduction of the NOMS Offender Management Model in 2006, the term 'offender manager' or 'case manager' rather than probation officer or probation services officer is often used to signify the person allocated overall responsibility for an offender's sentence. People about whom probation write reports or supervise are labelled 'offenders'. Critics of the term offender (for example, Weaver and McNeill 2007) argue that the label cements negative perceptions of people who have offended and may lead to a loss of belief in the possibility of reformation.

Assisting the court and assessing offenders

A major part of probation work is to assist magistrates' and Crown courts by preparing pre-sentence reports 'with a view to ... determining the most suitable method of dealing with an offender' (Criminal Justice Act 2003 s. 158 (1)(a) – www.legislation.gov.uk). When preparing a pre-sentence report, probation uses the Offender Assessment System (OASys) which was developed jointly by the prison service and probation. It is used to assess the likelihood of reoffending; the risk of serious harm should further offences occur; who is at risk of harm and under what circumstances; and an offender's ability and motivation to change their behaviour (Home Office 2002a). OASys produces a statistical prediction of the risk of reconviction but it cannot quantify the risk of future serious harm the person may pose to themselves or others. OASys also helps identify and classify offending related needs, including basic characteristics and cognitive behavioural problems. The completed assessment informs sentencing, risk management and decisions about intervention programmes.

Probation staff interview the offender, draw on material from criminal records and court papers, including victim statements, and take steps to verify the information the offender has provided. They may also contact other professionals to obtain information. For example, in a case relating to domestic abuse, it is important to find if the person has come to police notice for incidents relating to domestic abuse which did not proceed to prosecution. The result of an OASys assessment sometimes suggests a need for a further assessment (for example, in relation to mental health problems, domestic violence, sex offending, alcohol or drugs, or basic skills). These assessments may be carried out by probation staff or by other specialist professionals such as psychiatrists. Risks are categorised as being: risk of serious harm to others; risk to children; and/or risk to the individual offender.

Having completed this assessment, a pre-sentence report is prepared which sets out sources of information on which the report is based, an offence analysis to enable the court to understand why this person committed the offence, and the likely impact on the victim. An offender assessment then provides personal information about the offender relevant to understanding why the offence was committed and outlining any previous convictions, followed by a section assessing the offender's risk of harm to the public and likelihood of reoffending, concluding with information about sentencing options which might address the risks and needs identified.

Assessing and managing risk and working together with other professionals

Central tasks in probation work are the assessment of risk and the management of this risk in the community. Kempshall (2002) argues the emphasis on risk and protection reflects a general public anxiety about the dangers posed by offenders and leads to a defensive attitude to risk with an emphasis on precaution and prevention. The background to developments in interprofessional work to manage risk lies in the reporting of several high profile cases of offences committed by individuals already known to professionals in different agencies which drew attention to a critical need for effective interagency working. This led to the development of legislative frameworks to support interprofessional information sharing and risk management (for example, Sex Offenders Registration Act 1997, Children Act 2004 – www.legislation.gov.uk).

Multi Agency Public Protection Arrangements (MAPPA) require police and probation to liaise with the prison service and to negotiate the involvement of social services, local authority housing departments and the health service to work together in local MAPPA panels to protect the public from offenders thought to pose a serious risk. Exchange of confidential information between agencies must comply with the provisions of the Data Protection Act 1998 and the Human Rights Act 1998 (www.legislation.gov.uk). Information is shared in order to inform the risk assessment and to contribute to a joint plan to manage the risk. Social services are the lead agency for cases of risk to children and other vulnerable groups. Health service personnel provide advice about the appropriateness of health interventions, including mental health interventions. Housing departments advise on the safest housing options available for offenders returning to the community. The prison service provides information to probation and police about those who are being released. The majority of those considered by MAPPA are supervised by probation officers who are required to liaise with other agencies. The national IT system for management of people who pose a serious risk of harm to the public (VISoR) is used by the police, probation and prison service to share intelligence. Additionally, Multi Agency Risk Assessment Conferences (MARACs) address risk in cases of domestic abuse in order to provide a victim-focused coordinated community response. A number of evaluations of MARACs have been undertaken and results suggest they are saving lives and money (CAADA, 2010) when there are strong partnership links, strong leadership and good coordination of services (Home Office 2011).

CASE STUDY: pre-sentence work

The case study illustrates the process of interprofessional work in a case of domestic abuse.

(a) Arrest
The police arrested John, a white male in his early 30s, at his home. The victim of the offence was his partner Mary who had bruises to her neck and arms and a head cut. John was charged with an offence of Assault Occasioning Actual Bodily Harm and released on bail, with a condition not to return home or contact Mary. The police passed Mary's details to Noor, an Independent Domestic Violence Advisor. They also notified social services because children were present when John was arrested.

(b) Women's safety work
Noor (the Independent Domestic Violence Advisor) immediately contacted Mary to offer support and learned that Mary was pregnant and had two young children, aged three and six. Noor completed a severity of abuse and a risk assessment checklist (CAADA 2009) with Mary and asked her to sign a Confidentiality and Information Agreement (CAADA 2012). Noor explained that she would be sharing information with other services so that agencies could act together to promote safety for Mary and her children. Mary explained that John had been violent and abusive to her for several years, especially when he had been drinking, prevented her from seeing her mother and other family members, and had recently twice attempted to strangle her. She had thought about leaving but was frightened as John said he would kill her if she left him. Noor advised Mary to contact the police immediately if she felt threatened and they discussed how she might keep herself and children safe. Noor gave Mary information about services (such as panic alarms), discussed some of her legal options and where to get additional advice and support advising Mary to share her concerns with her doctor and community midwife. Together they drew up an Individualised Safety and

Support Action Plan for Mary and her children. Noor explained that she would be referring Mary to the MARAC giving her a leaflet about this explaining that she would support Mary during this process. Mary's situation was reviewed by the next MARAC. The local agencies present (including the police, social services, health and probation) shared their information about the family and drew up a risk-focused, coordinated safety plan. The police agreed to advise operational units to respond as a priority to any reports of incidents at Mary's address.

(c) A referral from court

John appeared at the magistrates' court and pleaded guilty. He had one previous conviction for assault (one year ago) and a conviction for drinking and driving (two years ago). His case was adjourned for a pre-sentence report. John was released on bail to live with his mother with a condition not to contact Mary. A probation officer, Nina, was assigned to write the report. In discussion with the police community safety unit, Nina discovered that the police had responded to 15 domestic call-outs in the past year.

(d) The assessment of the offender

Nina reviewed the court papers, probation records and the police information. Nina then interviewed John using the OASys assessment form and the SARA, a domestic assault risk assessment tool (Kropp and Hart 2000). John admitted assaulting Mary but maintained that he had only been abusive to her once. He blamed Mary for provoking him saying he would never be violent to Mary again and that he wanted the relationship to continue. The OASys assessment tool indicated factors related to relationships and alcohol use as key areas associated with risk of reoffending. Nina assessed John as posing a high risk of violence to Mary. She told John that she was considering proposing a community sentence with a condition that he attends a domestic abuse programme and undertakes alcohol counselling and includes these details in the pre-sentence report.

QUESTIONS

- How many different types of professionals have been involved with John, Mary and their children since John was arrested?
- What are the main risks in this case? Who is at risk and why? What might increase the risks? What might reduce the risks?

In your answers you will have identified that professionals from at least five different agencies will have been involved with Mary and John and their children. There are probably quite a few more. Did you consider the midwife and the doctor? With so many professionals working with the family, one thing which might increase risk is if professionals say something negative to John about his behaviour which they have learned from Mary. Having different professionals working with John and Mary is one way to reduce this risk.

Working with offenders subject to community sentences and licences

The *Practice Framework* (MJ/NOMS 2011) sets out a consistent approach to practice to deliver offender management services in the community. The acronym ASPIRE is used to describe the standard range of work governed by the National Standards framework: Assessment; Sentence Plan; Implement; Review; and Evaluate. Probation and rehabilitation services are required to secure offender compliance with the requirements of their sentence and to take enforcement action in cases of failure to comply, normally by taking offenders back to court.

The *Practice Framework* encourages more practitioner use of discretion and judgement than previous standards, arguing that by reducing prescription, innovation will be encouraged. Emphasis is placed on providing an individualised service in which workers 'do the right thing with the right individual in the right way at the right time' (MJ/NOMS 2011: 3) in order to reduce reoffending and protect the public. Research on desistance from offending (Maruna and LeBel 2010, Weaver and McNeill 2007) suggests that a positive professional response is essential to stopping reoffending. Practice is guided by the risk-need-responsivity model (Bonta and Andrews 2010) which means targeting interventions at those who are assessed to pose the most risk; focusing interventions at needs associated with the person's offending; and working with people in a way which encourages full participation taking into account identity and diversity. The intervention plan (supervision plan) must include how identified risks are going to be addressed and may include multiagency arrangements such as referral to MAPPA or MARAC and liaison with social services or mental health professionals.

Direct work with offenders to reduce offending is based on evidence of effectiveness of interventions. Emphasis is placed on developing a community-based multimodal approach to intervention that is skills-oriented and models pro-social behaviour. A range of individual and group work programmes (such as cognitive behavioural programmes, domestic abuse programmes and community sex offenders programmes) are available for offenders to undertake as part of their programme of rehabilitation and one or more of these will normally be a required element of their sentence. Common themes in all programmes are enabling offenders to accept full responsibility for their offending; enhancing understanding of thinking patterns, feelings and behaviours which can lead to offending; examining what created opportunities to offend and what he or she can do in the future to avoid this; raising awareness of the effects on victims as offenders can use thinking errors to convince themselves their behaviour is acceptable; learning to recognise high-risk situations; and providing opportunities to practise steps to take to avoid further offending.

Working together to support victims of crime

Victim services and support aim to ensure victims' interests become central to the Criminal Justice System and probation has to adhere to *The Code of Practice for Victims of Crime* (CJS 2006). Government policy aims to develop a national framework for collaborative working among agencies within the Criminal Justice System to promote victims' rights and safety. A clear focus is kept on the effects of crime on victims with the aim of requiring offenders to face up to the impact of their actions on others. In a domestic abuse case, a referral will be made to a specialist women's safety worker as part of an integrated approach to provide support to victims of domestic abuse and their children. Women's safety workers liaise with other agencies to provide support to women and children living in contexts of domestic abuse. They offer a continuing service to women victims following sentence, helping women access specialist services, such as legal advice, refuge provision, children's services and housing advice. While the needs of women and children are often similar, the safety of children is always paramount. An important point to note here is that when there are concerns about the safety of the child, confidentiality is limited and concerns must be reported to social services. Information provided by women victims is never disclosed directly to offenders as this may increase the risk to women and children.

CASE STUDY continued

John is sentenced to a Community Order for two years with requirements that he attends the domestic abuse programme, addresses his alcohol problem and undertakes 100 hours unpaid work. John is given an appointment at court to report to Jim, the practitioner responsible for his supervision, to start his programme of supervision and rehabilitation. Jim also refers Mary to the Women's Safety Service. Jim explains the requirements of the order to John and what will happen if he fails to keep appointments. Jim reviews the pre-sentence report and OASys assessment and draws up a supervision plan with John. He is also given an appointment to meet with the Community Payback Service to start unpaid work as part of his sentence.

John tells Jim that he has moved back home with Mary, he has promised to stop drinking and never to assault her again. Jim asks him to identify what steps he plans to take to stop behaving abusively and makes an appointment for alcohol counselling to start the following week. After the meeting Jim lets the Police Community Safety Unit, probation, social services and the Women's Safety Service know that John has moved home again.

Jenny, a women's safety worker from a community agency working in partnership with probation, contacts Mary, confirms John's story, discusses safety planning and also ensures that Mary understands that there is no guarantee that the programme will be a success. Jenny offers to keep Mary informed about John's attendance on the domestic abuse programme and advises her to contact the police immediately if she feels under threat.

John attends the domestic abuse group work programme for the next 30 weeks. He also has regular meetings with the alcohol counsellor and he undertakes unpaid work. Jim receives weekly reports about John from the domestic abuse group work programme, and feedback from unpaid work and the alcohol counsellor. During this period Jenny keeps in touch with Mary and lets Jim know about any concerns.

John meets with Jim once a month to review his progress.

Review the information provided in the two extracts of the case study and consider the following questions:

- What professionals and agencies will John and Mary be in contact with during the period John is on a Community Order?
- What concerns or risks can you identify in this situation and how should this information be shared?
- Who should take responsibility for sharing information?
- What problems can you identify about sharing information in this case?
- What benefits might come from sharing information and working together?

In your answers to these questions, you will have realised that more agency personnel are now involved with John and Mary. The Independent Domestic Violence Advisor will have withdrawn and her role is taken over by the Women's Safety Service. Did you consider that a risk may be now that John had returned home, Mary may not feel as able to access support? Who do you think would be the lead agency in this case?

Conclusion: working together interprofessionally – challenges and visions

This chapter has highlighted the need for coordination between agencies working with offenders and for collaboration between probation and rehabilitation services and other professionals in order to protect the public, to reduce reoffending, and to work with victims of crime. It is increasingly recognised that effective practice to reduce reoffending and to rehabilitate offenders requires the development of purposeful working relationships between agencies and professionals.

Contributing to local crime and disorder strategies and being part of Multiagency Public Protection Arrangements are requirements for probation. The potential of a coordinated approach can be glimpsed in the efforts of active and purposeful networking of individuals from different agencies in relation to working with domestic abuse. New initiatives include probation and social workers providing programmes jointly for fathers where there has been domestic abuse in the family – The Caring Dads programme (Scott, Francis, Crooks and Kelly 2006). Legislation, protocols and procedures for interagency working legitimate and require such contact. Effective collaborative working requires professionals to learn about each other's perspectives, priorities, responsibilities and remit. It also requires probation to share information with, and recognise the contribution of other professionals. Professionals working together need to recognise power relationships which can result in conflicts of interest and nurture interprofessional relationships. Trust needs to be earned by principled conduct and pro-active communication to promote understanding and to acknowledge, address and resolve any difficulties that may arise. Forging productive collaborative relationships requires significant investment of time, energy and human resources. The potential returns on such investment are high in terms of providing effective services to offenders, victims and communities.

RECOMMENDED READING

■ Canton R. (2011) *Probation: Working with Offenders*. Abingdon: Routledge.
■ Gelsthorpe L. and Morgan R. (eds) (2007) *Handbook of Probation*. Cullompton: Willan.
■ McNeill F., Raynor P. and Trotter C. (2010) *Offender Supervision: New Directions in Theory, Research and Practice*. Abingdon: Willan.

References

Allen R. and Hough M. (2007) Community penalties, sentencers, the media and public opinion. In Gelsthorpe L. and Morgan R. (eds), *Handbook of Probation*. Cullompton: Willan, pp. 565–601.

Bonta J. and Andrews D. (2010) Viewing offender assessment and rehabilitation through the lens of the risk-needs-responsivity model. In McNeill F., Raynor P. and Trotter C. (2010) *Offender Supervision: New Directions in Theory, Research and Practice*. Abingdon: Willan, pp 19–40.

CAADA (2009) *Domestic Abuse, Stalking and 'Honour'-based Violence (DASH) Risk Identification Checklist*. www.caada.org.uk. Accessed June 2012.

CAADA (2010) *Saving Lives. Saving Money: MARACS and High Risk Domestic Abuse*. www.caada.org.uk. Accessed November 2012.

CAADA (2012) *Case Management Pack for IDVAs to Use in their Day-to-Day Role*. www.caada.org.uk. Accessed June 2012.

Canton R. (2011) *Probation: Working with Offenders*. Abingdon: Routledge.

Casey L. (2008) *Engaging Communities in Fighting Crime: A Review (Casey Report)*. London: Cabinet Office.

CJS (Criminal Justice System) (2006) *Code of Practice for Victims of Crime*. www.cps.gov.uk. Accessed November 2012.

GB (Great Britain) Probation of Offenders Act 1907. www.probation.ie. Accessed June 2013.

GB (2013) *Transforming Rehabilitation: A Strategy for Reform Presented to Parliament by the Lord Chancellor and Secretary of State for Justice by Command of Her Majesty*. London: The Stationery Office.

Gelsthorpe L. (2007) Probation values and human rights. In Gelsthorpe L. and Morgan R. (eds), *Handbook of Probation*. Cullompton: Willan, pp. 485–517.

Home Office (2001) *Probation Circular 25/2001*. London: Home Office.

Home Office (2002a) *Offender Assessment System OASys User Manual*. London: Home Office.

Home Office (2011) *Supporting High Risk Victims of Domestic Abuse: A Review of Multi-Agency Risk Assessment Conferences (MARACs)*. www.homeoffice.gov.uk. Accessed November 2012.

Jansson K. (2008) *British Crime Survey: Measuring Crime for 25 Years*. London: Home Office.

Kempshall H. (2002) Risk, public protection and justice. In Ward D., Scott J. and Lacey M. (eds), *Probation: Working for Justice* (2nd edn). Oxford: Oxford University Press, pp. 95–110.

Kropp R. and Hart S. (2000) The Spousal Assault Risk Assessment (SARA) Guide: reliability and validity in adult male offenders. *Law and Human Behavior*, **24**(1): 101–18.

Maruna S. and King A. (2008) Selling the public on probation: beyond the bib. *Probation Journal* **55**(4): 337–51.

Maruna S. and LeBel T. (2010) The desistance paradigm in correctional practice: from programmes to lives. In McNeill F., Raynor P. and Trotter C. (2010) *Offender Supervision: New Directions in Theory, Research and Practice*. Abingdon: Willan, pp. 65–88.

MJ/NOMS (Ministry of Justice/National Offender Management Service) (2011) *The Practice Framework: National Standards for the Management of Offenders*. London: MJ.

Nellis M (2002) Community justice and the new probation service. *Howard Journal* **41**(1): 59–86.

NOMS (National Offender Management Service) (2011) *Values Statement.* www.justice.gov.uk. Accessed June 2012.

Scott K., Francis K., Crooks C. and Kelly T. (2006). *Caring Dads: Helping Fathers Value their Children.* Victoria, BC: Trafford.

Weaver B. and McNeill F. (2007) *Giving Up Crime: Directions for Policy.* Edinburgh: Scottish Consortium for Crime and Criminal Justice.

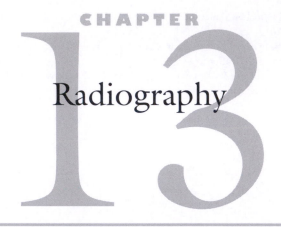

CHAPTER 13

Radiography

Jan Chianese, Karen Dunmall and Ken Holmes

Introduction

This chapter explores the roles of radiographers in the diagnosis and management of a patient diagnosed with cancer. A case study is used to show how radiographers work as part of the interprofessional team when assisting a patient during their journey through diagnosis and treatment. The chapter outlines existing and developing practices of radiographers and illustrates some aspects of role boundaries when working collaboratively.

Radiography

The title of radiographer encompasses two distinct professions each with its own title protected by the Health and Care Professions Council (HCPC): diagnostic imaging radiographer and therapeutic radiographer. The diagnostic imaging radiographer is primarily involved with the production of images used to aid diagnosis, while the therapeutic radiographer is involved with the delivery of ionising radiation for the treatment of cancers. To work in the United Kingdom a radiographer must have completed an approved educational programme and be registered with the HCPC. A radiography practitioner can develop specialist skills to become an advanced practitioner and then, after further education and training, a consultant practitioner. The career development framework for radiography also includes another tier of workers, assistant practitioners, who are not HCPC registered. Assistant practitioners can undertake non-complex imaging examinations or assist therapeutic radiographers in radiotherapy treatments and associated procedures (SCoR 2007a).

Both diagnostic imaging and therapeutic radiographers require a three-year full-time (or equivalent) programme of study in preparation for registration and subsequent practice. Generally, the educational programmes comprise equal time spent in the hospital environment and in the university. The clinical components require specific placements in appropriate hospital departments exposing students to patient care provided by a range of multidisciplinary teams.

Working with radiation

X-rays and gamma radiation are known as ionising radiations and can cause damage to cells and tissues. Doses of ionising radiation, whether naturally occurring or man-made, have the potential to cause cancers although the additional cancer risk from exposure to low doses is effectively undetectable in the general population (HPA 2008). The use of ionising radiation is controlled by European legislation under the Ionising Radiations (Medical Exposure) Regulations (IR(ME)R 2000) which sets out the education and training required for radiography practice. In addition, Regulations 11 and 12 determine the role of practitioners within radiology and radiotherapy services (IR(ME)R 2000). The Ionising Radiation Regulations 1999 (www.legislation. gov.uk) set out guidelines for the health and safety of those working with ionising radiations. Health care professionals working in this environment need to be able to understand and communicate the risks of ionising radiation in a way that is both clear and reassuring to patients.

The role of the diagnostic imaging radiographer

Diagnostic radiographers play a pivotal role in the imaging of patients leading to the diagnosing of disease. The main methods of imaging undertaken by diagnostic radiographers involve the use of X-rays. Diagnostic radiographers are required to produce high quality images of the body. The successful production of a diagnostic image relies on the ability of the radiographer to communicate effectively with the patient (the term 'patient' is used here to be synonymous with 'service user' or 'client', depending on the service accessed along a person's treatment and care pathway). The radiographer will need to discuss the radiographic examination and its consequences, answer questions about the procedure and try to put the patient at ease (Springett and Dunmall 2009). This will include explaining the balance of risks versus benefits of the examination. In addition to working in the general imaging departments found in most hospitals, diagnostic radiographers work in accident and emergency departments, specialist centres, hospital wards using portable imaging equipment, and in community departments. In these different environments, diagnostic radiographers work alongside radiologists (consultant doctors who specialise in radiology), nurses, technicians and other medical staff. Radiographers can specialise in other imaging modalities using either ionising radiation (for example, computerised tomography and nuclear medicine) or non-ionising imaging modalities (for example, ultrasound and magnetic resonance imaging). There is increasing use of imaging modalities in the radiotherapy field to image patients in respect of targeting their cancer for treatment. This development of imaging modalities has led to collaborative working in terms of a cross-over between diagnostic and treatment domains, where imaging resources may be shared and therapeutic radiographers begin to develop some of the skills associated with diagnostic imaging.

The role of the therapeutic radiographer

Unlike diagnostic imaging, radiotherapy makes therapeutic use of the destructive power of high-energy ionising radiation to kill cancer cells in a precise and controlled manner. Therapeutic radiographers work in oncology departments (where tumours are studied and treated) sited mainly either in purpose-built hospitals, or in specialist units within large general hospitals. Radiotherapy is a treatment used to eradicate cancer cells or to relieve symptoms of advanced cancer (palliative treatment). Palliation can mean, for example, alleviating pain from cancer spread to bone or relieving breathlessness caused by lung cancer. Radiotherapy is also used alongside surgery, cytotoxic chemotherapy or hormone therapy in the treatment of cancers. The most common type of radiotherapy equipment is the linear accelerator, which produces photon energies in the order of millions of electron volts compared to the mere thousands produced by general diagnostic X-ray machines.

Therapeutic radiographers also work with diagnostic imaging equipment to produce images for the purpose of planning radiotherapy treatments. Radiotherapy departments may use simulators to mimic the movements of the linear accelerator and this enables the therapeutic radiographer to visualise the potential pathway of a therapy beam prior to the start of treatment. Radiotherapy departments will have either a computerised tomography (CT) scanner or a CT simulator for radiotherapy planning. Modern linear accelerators have the facility to produce images while treatment is taking place and these snapshot images help reinforce checks needed to verify that the target area of the cancer is being treated. With this technology, ongoing image-guided radiotherapy can be used to adapt and alter treatment targets according to changes in tumour growth, changes in patient shape, or to adjust to internal organ movement.

CASE STUDY: Thandie Washington

Thandie Washington, a 50-year-old full-time working mother of two teenage children, received her first invitation for a routine screening mammogram from her general practitioner (GP) surgery. During the mammogram, the assistant diagnostic imaging practitioner explains to Thandie that it is necessary to get firm pressure on her breast tissue between the plates of the machine to get a technically satisfactory image as this will help to distinguish abnormal from normal tissue. Knowing the reasons for the procedure and knowing also that it may be slightly uncomfortable will help Thandie prepare for the examination. The examination is over in a few minutes and Thandie is informed that she will receive the results by letter. Two weeks later Thandie is worried because she has been recalled for a second mammogram. Her husband, Shane, has decided to accompany her.

========================= **QUESTION** =========================

▓ What concerns might Thandie have about being recalled for a second mammogram?

Thandie is likely to be anxious and frightened by being recalled as she may think it means a diagnosis of cancer. She may be wondering what this might mean to her and her family, and she may be thinking through a number of different scenarios and outcomes. She may consider putting off making any plans until she has been for her second visit.

Thandie will have received some information with her initial invitation which she will be able to refer to when she receives her recall letter. This is intended to alleviate her anxieties (NHSBSP 2012). Thandie may access information and support via her GP or practice nurse prior to the second appointment. She might also access online support agencies recommended by a health care professional such as NHS Choices (www.nhs.uk) and the NHS Breast Screening Programme (www.cancerscreening.nhs.uk). Information is available in various formats to meet the needs of people who might have, for example, learning disabilities, a hearing impairment or poor literacy skills.

========================= **QUESTION** =========================

▓ How might the diagnostic radiographer respond to Thandie's concerns when she arrives at the clinic?

The radiographer will try to reassure Thandie by reinforcing the information provided in the Breast Screening pamphlet (NHSBSP 2012). The radiographer will explain that as this was her first screening episode there are no previous images to compare to and assess what is normal for her.

========================= **QUESTION** =========================

▓ What might be the dilemmas for the breast screening team in giving information prior to a definitive result?

The team will recognise that there is a strong possibility of a diagnosis of cancer but will need to balance this with the possibility of a false positive result. Thus the team will refrain from giving this information until all clinical tests have been completed. This may present some challenges to the health care professionals in matching their non-verbal language to their verbal communication.

CASE STUDY continued

Thandie has been recalled because of irregularities in the image taken on her first visit. An irregularity can appear as a result of the anatomical position of overlapping breast tissue leading to difficulty in distinguishing between normal and abnormal tissue. Under these circumstances a registered diagnostic imaging radiographer will be able to adjust the technology in order to obtain a less ambiguous image. Thus on her second visit, Thandie is seen by Catriona (a registered diagnostic imaging radiographer) so that images beyond the scope of the assistant practitioner can be taken and assessed for clarity. A second visit usually takes place at a one-stop clinic where a breast care team would be ready to support Thandie through the examination and refer her, if necessary, for further procedures. Catriona tells Thandie that the image will be processed while she waits in the department and she will then be able to discuss the results with a member of the breast care team. Catriona ensures that Thandie's questions about the procedure are answered before taking the X-ray image.

In order to reduce the number of errors in diagnoses all images are reviewed independently by two members of the diagnostic imaging team (this will be either two radiographers or a radiographer and a radiologist) who then compare results before a diagnosis is made. After obtaining a suitable image Catriona identifies an area of microcalcification seen as small white specks on the image and as a potential indicator of cancer. She passes her report to the consultant doctor who confirms that the image is strongly suggestive of breast cancer.

The breast care team normally includes a specialist breast care nurse, a radiographer and a doctor or consultant radiographer. Communicating the results of a mammogram is an important part of the role of the breast care team as each member is skilled in communication and able to answer questions about prognosis, treatment options, and further imaging procedures. The leading clinician (who will be either a doctor or a consultant radiographer) explains to Thandie the requirement for further diagnostic tests. Following the results of the tests, it would be possible to tell Thandie whether the diagnosis is benign or malignant.

Unfortunately in this case the disease is malignant and the leading clinician informs Thandie of the diagnosis. Shane is included in the discussion and the breast care specialist nurse is present to support Thandie and Shane. A diagnosis of cancer is life changing so it is likely they will need some time to digest the news and they will be provided with material (perhaps in written or DVD format) about the diagnosis, prognosis and treatment options to enable them to review the information at any time after the consultation.

Treatment will depend on the exact location of the cancer in Thandie's breast, on whether or not there is metastatic spread, and on the specific cell types involved. Most patients will undergo radionuclide imaging in an attempt to detect metastatic spread from the primary cancer before it is visible on plain radiographs. In this instance further tests reveal that the cancer is confined to Thandie's breast.

Following discussion with the oncologist (a consultant doctor specialising in cancer) about her treatment options, Thandie decides on surgery followed by a course of radiotherapy. The aim of this particular type of surgery (commonly known as 'lumpectomy') is to remove the cancer together with some surrounding tissue, while the aim of the radiotherapy treatment is to eradicate any remaining cancer cells around the operation site. Thandie will be supported from the point of diagnosis throughout her surgery by the breast care team.

The breast care nurse will have seen Thandie and her husband prior to her surgery in order to discuss how surgery may affect her body shape and her body image. The surgeon will have discussed with Thandie the prospect of reconstructive surgery once she has completed the treatment. Thandie opts for some reconstructive surgery following her radiotherapy offered as a result of discussions at the multidisciplinary team meeting. In the meantime she discusses with the breast care nurse how to look after her skin during the radiotherapy treatment and the types of clothes that will help her to remain comfortable with her appearance. The breast care nurse may offer Thandie a temporary prosthesis to wear following surgery. Shane is keen to be involved in the discussions in order to support Thandie during this time when she feels vulnerable and anxious. She is worried that she may lose her hair as she has heard that this is a side effect of cancer treatments. The nurse tells Thandie that hair loss is a common side effect of cytotoxic chemotherapy but when receiving radiotherapy hair loss is restricted to the localised area of treatment so Thandie will only lose body hair on her skin at the treatment site. Thandie is also worried about what radiotherapy will entail and so the breast care nurse liaises with the therapeutic radiography team to organise a familiarisation visit to the radiotherapy department. During the familiarisation visit Thandie is shown around the department and is able to see the machines and rooms where she will have treatment. She takes advantage of the opportunity to discuss her concerns regarding treatment with Lara, one of the therapeutic radiographers.

Following successful lumpectomy to remove the cancer, an appointment is made for Thandie to attend the pre-treatment suite at the radiotherapy department in the oncology centre. The pre-treatment preparation involves use of equipment such as a simulator or CT scanner. This visit allows the radiotherapy team to plan the first part of the treatment and provides Thandie with another opportunity to ask questions.

Lara (the therapeutic radiographer who Thandie met during her familiarisation visit) takes Thandie through the process step-by-step, answering her questions and making arrangements for her first treatment appointment. Lara explains the process of the simulation and the treatment to follow. Thandie has many questions but may not understand all aspects of the treatment because she is likely to be nervous (Brennan 2004) and because there is a lot of information to absorb. As Thandie is very anxious about starting treatment she has brought Shane with her and has asked if he can sit in during the talk with the radiographer. Shane is pleased to be included in the process as this will help them as they explain to other family members what Thandie will be going through during treatment. Support from Shane and the family will be invaluable to Thandie as she progresses through the treatment and beyond.

Lara helps Thandie assume the correct position on the simulator couch and explains the need for Thandie to position her arms in particular ways while images are taken. The pre-treatment process involves a team consisting of the oncologist, medical physics technicians, physicists and therapeutic radiographers. Lara reinforces the information given at the beginning of the procedure, answers Thandie's questions, and takes her to meet a member of the team on the unit where she will receive treatment.

A team of therapeutic radiographers operate the linear accelerator that delivers radiotherapy in the treatment room. Long-term exposure to the high energy levels of the radiation used for radiotherapy is harmful so the radiographers cannot stay in the room with Thandie during treatment. Gaining Thandie's trust will help the radiographer to ensure that Thandie maintains the position she was in for her pre-treatment planning; this ensures that the treatment beam is always directed to the correct part of her body.

Therapeutic radiographers are involved in the process of gaining informed consent for treatment. This will include reminding Thandie of the potential effects and possible (early and late) side effects of radiotherapy as well as how to look after herself during treatment (Robinson 2007). Once Thandie has been given the information and has had the opportunity to ask questions, she will be asked to sign a consent form for the radiotherapy to begin. Because the team will see her each day of the week they are well placed to monitor the reaction of Thandie's skin together with any other side effects. They also work with other health care professionals, for example: the specialist breast care nurse, to advise on skin care, the dietician to advise on diet, and the oncologist to prescribe medications to minimise, relieve or treat side effects. Consultant and advanced radiotherapy practitioners with the appropriate specialism will be able to offer counselling or to prescribe particular medications to help with side effects.

On the first day of treatment, Anusha (a therapeutic radiographer who is part of Thandie's treatment team) introduces herself and explains to Thandie what will happen at the start and during treatment. Anusha takes Thandie into the treatment room where she finds that the process is similar to the one she experienced in the simulator. Once the lights are dimmed in the room the treatment team ensure the radiotherapy beams are lined up accurately by using light lasers to help define the treatment area. The printed computerised plan produced by the planning team of physicists and radiotherapy dosimetrists reproduces the measurements that coincide with the surface anatomy of Thandie's body and depicts the pathways and dose distribution of the radiation beams. A light beam shines on Thandie's chest to simulate the position of the radiation beam. (Some small diodes are taped onto Thandie's chest to double check dose measurements on the first day once the treatment has taken place.) Once the team is satisfied that Thandie is positioned correctly and that she knows how to contact them should she feel uncomfortable during the treatment, the radiographers leave the room to switch on the machine and Thandie's radiotherapy begins. Thandie attends the radiotherapy department for treatment daily between Monday and Friday for five weeks, and gets to know the team who are responsible for her treatment.

QUESTION

■ If you were undergoing radiotherapy treatment what skills and qualities would you expect the radiotherapy team to demonstrate?

We expect that you will have identified some of the following as skills and qualities helpful to members of the radiotherapy team when working with patients undergoing radiotherapy treatment: effective communication skills, caring and empathetic attitude, professionalism, attention to detail and accuracy. These skills and qualities are important in order to help patients during treatment regimes. Can you identify why they are necessary? Did you identify other skills or qualities that might be important? Can you say why you think they are important?

QUESTION

■ Why do you think communication between different professionals working with Thandie during her treatment is important?

Delivery of treatments involving radiation requires accurate information to be communicated between health care professionals. Patients need to be confident that their treatment pathway is clear to those involved so there is no room for error in information sharing. It is essential that Thandie and Shane have multidisciplinary support to ensure that the journey from diagnosis to treatment is seamless.

QUESTION

■ What might help or hinder communication between professionals in this sort of situation? (Think about this in particular in terms of practical issues and staff attitudes.)

Barriers to effective communication may result from entrenched hierarchies within and between staff groups, leading to non-sharing of information. Pressure of time in a busy department may lead to information not being clearly relayed between members of the team and this may open up the possibility of errors being made. Staff members may be located in different places at different times and may not give the same priority to the exchange of information gathered at different points in the pathway.

Cancer is one of the most common diseases in the Western world and as it is a disease associated with older age, the workload in radiotherapy departments will rise in conjunction with the demands of an increasingly ageing population. Technological developments in imaging and radiotherapy equipment are constantly evolving, leading to more cancers being diagnosed and treated successfully with a concomitant increase in the number of people living with cancer (DH 2007).

There are a growing number of initiatives focusing on the standards of care for cancer patients and the timely delivery of treatment. Cancer services provision should be patient-centred seamless care undertaken by an interprofessional team (NCAT 2009) and the National Cancer Patient Forum (NCAT 2010) provides users with an opportunity to have a voice in the development of services for people with cancer. Therapeutic radiographers need to have knowledge of treatments (such as surgery and chemotherapy) that are delivered alongside radiotherapy as well as knowledge of the role of other health care professionals involved in the delivery and aftercare of treatments. Liaison with oncologists, nurse teams (specifically oncology nurses), medical physicists, health care assistants and technicians is often required on a daily basis in radiotherapy and oncology departments. This may extend to involve other health care and social care professionals, as therapeutic radiographers are often the first point of contact for many outpatients receiving treatment lasting several weeks.

Role development in radiography

Development of the four-tier structure from assistant practitioner through to consultant radiographer set out by the Department of Health (DH 2003) laid out the banding of roles and responsibilities in the health care environment for diagnostic imaging and therapeutic radiography services. The scope of practice for each of these four roles is set by the Society and College of Radiographers (SCoR 2007a, b), and by the HCPC (2009). Becoming an advanced or consultant practitioner usually involves further education and training related to the specific skills set required; for example, a postgraduate certificate in mammography or a Master's degree in specialist practice. For suitably qualified diagnostic radiographers, this will mean having discretion to perform additional images, undertake diagnostic examinations, and report on the images produced from these procedures within set protocols. Consultant or advanced diagnostic imaging radiographers may be responsible for their own patient caseload or list; for example, a list of patients for barium study examinations that would have been previously undertaken by a radiologist. For therapeutic radiographers, the role can extend within the clinical oncology setting to develop specialist areas of work previously outside their remit. This may include running their own caseload of, for example, brachytherapy patients or leading a clinic to review patients undergoing treatment, and pre-scribing medication within a defined remit (SCoR 2009).

Conclusion

Patients attending for diagnostic imaging and radiotherapy rely on their healthcare professionals to deliver a caring, safe and accurate quality service. Radiographers undertake specialist education and training for their individual professions but actively work in interprofessional teams to produce holistic patient-centred care. Radiographers work within a specific scope of practice; however, there are increasing opportunities for role extensions in both techno-logical and patient-focused areas.

RECOMMENDED READING

- Cameron J.L., Blyth C.M. and Kirby A.S. (2008) An audit of a radiotherapy review clinic for breast cancer patients: a multi-disciplinary approach. *Journal of Radiotherapy in Practice* **7**(4): 233–9.
- DH (Department of Health) (2007) *Radiotherapy: Developing a World Class Service for England. Report to Ministers from National Radiotherapy Advisory Group.* www.dh.gov.uk. Accessed February 2013.
- Easton S. (ed.) *An Introduction to Radiography.* London: Churchill Livingstone.
- Mathers S.A., McKenzie G.A. and Robertson E.M. (2013) 'It was daunting': experience of women with a diagnosis of breast cancer attending for breast imaging. *Radiography* **19**(2): 156–63.
- Society and College of Radiographers website *www.sor.org*

References

Brennan J. (2004) *Cancer in Context: A Practical Guide to Supportive Care*. Oxford: Oxford University Press.

DH (Department of Health) (2003) *Radiography Skills Mix: A Report on the Four-tier Service Delivery Model*. London: DH.

DH (2007) *Radiotherapy: Developing a World Class Service for England. Report to Ministers from National Radiotherapy Advisory Group*. www.dh.gov.uk. Accessed February 2013.

HCPC (Health and Care Professions Council) (2009) *Standards of Proficiency – Radiographers*. London: HCPC.

HPA (Health Protection Agency) (2008) *The Estimation of Cancer Risk at Low Doses*. www.hpa. org.uk. Accessed February 2013.

Ionising Radiation (Medical Exposure) Regulations (2000). www.doh.gov.uk. Accessed February 2013.

NCAT (National Cancer Action Team) (2009) *Multidisciplinary Team Members' Views about MDT Working: Results from a Survey Commissioned by the National Cancer Action Team*. www. ncat.nhs.uk. Accessed February 2013.

NCAT (2010) The National Cancer Patient Forum. www.ncat.nhs.uk. Accessed February 2013.

NHSBSP (NHS Breast Screening Programme) (2012) *NHS Breast Screening*. www.cancerscreening.nhs.uk. Accessed February 2013.

Robinson K.S. (2007) The consent process in radiotherapy. *Journal of Radiotherapy in Practice* 6(4): 211–16.

SCoR (Society and College of Radiographers) (2007a) *The Scope of Practice of Assistant Practitioners in Radiotherapy*. London: SCoR.

SCoR (2007b) *Learning and Development Framework for Clinical Imaging and Oncology*. London: SCoR.

SCoR (2009) *Scope of Practice*. London: SCoR.

Springett G. and Dunmall K. (2009) Communication. In Easton S. (ed.), *An Introduction to Radiography*. London: Churchill Livingstone, pp. 23–40.

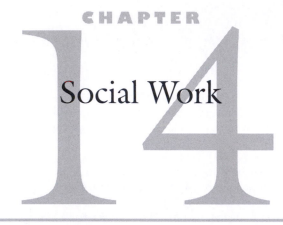

Social Work

Adrian Vatcher and Karen Jones

Introduction

This chapter offers a brief overview of social work and its historical development, outlines the nature of modern social work and offers an illustration of
the way in which social workers contribute to interprofessional working.
Most social workers in England and Wales are employed by local authorities, voluntary organisations, health trusts and most recently, 'social enterprises'. Social workers have a key role in meeting local authorities'
obligations to provide information, advice and services to support children,
young people, disabled adults and older people at risk or in need. Though
these services were once organised into single Social Services Departments
it is now more usual for services for children and young people, and for disabled adults and older people to be provided by a variety of separate organisations.

Social workers are concerned with addressing need and risk. In order
to do this, they work closely with a range of other professions including
housing officers, teachers, police, occupational therapists, psychologists,
health professionals and care workers. Social workers may be based in locality
offices, day centres, residential care homes, hospitals or community projects
in teams consisting mainly of social workers or in multiprofessional teams.
The role of the social worker therefore varies according to context. However,
the case study in this chapter seeks to draw out some key practice themes, of
relevance to any setting.

Defining social work

Social work is defined internationally as promoting:

> social change, problem solving in human relationships and the empowerment and liberation of people to enhance well-being. Utilising theories of human behaviour and social systems, social work intervenes at the points where people interact with their environments. Principles of human rights and social justice are fundamental to social work.
>
> (IASSW/IFSW 2001: 1)

This definition covers a wide range of practices in different social and political contexts across the world. The commentary accompanying it highlights the role of the professional as working 'in solidarity with those who are disadvantaged' (IASSW/IFSW 2001: 1) in alleviating poverty, promoting social inclusion and identifying a range of interventions from working with individuals to involvement in social policy.

In England the College of Social Work provides a more publicly accessible, but less politically ambitious definition of the contribution of social work:

> Social work is the 'safety net' of society. Trained and qualified social workers intervene into private and/or family life in order to:
> - protect individuals from harm to themselves or to others
> - promote human development and security, social inclusion and participation across the lifespan.
>
> (CSW 2009: 1)

Whatever the formal definition, social work practice encompasses a range of activities from individual counselling, through arranging support and services, to political action:

- Listening, communicating and counselling – engaging with service users and carers to build trusting relationships.
- Giving information, signposting and being an advocate – enabling people to recognise and secure their entitlements and on occasions, speak directly on their behalf.
- Assessment of needs – exploring people's needs with them to identify ways of addressing the difficulties they are experiencing.
- Acting as a gatekeeper of resources – assessing social needs and deciding whether clients are eligible for a service.
- Coordinating services for people with complex needs.
- Assessment of risk and making decisions to intervene, within a legal framework, to protect children and vulnerable adults.
- Working in the community to address circumstances creating social problems (Adams, Dominelli and Payne 2009, Coulshed and Orme 1998, Trevithick 2012).

A complex activity

There is potentially a high degree of overlap between the responsibilities, knowledge, and skills of social workers and those of other professions. The distinctive contribution of social workers in any given situation will depend partly on the agency in which they are working and partly on the particular interests and skills of the staff they are working with.

It is important to recognise that social work is inherently political as it takes place only as a collectively organised response to public concern about complex social problems. This means that while social workers may have a highly developed sense of what their knowledge and skills are and what they are for, they can only stake their claim to power and authority through appeal to some collective conception of the general good – political, religious or otherwise – and an assertion that they know how it might best be achieved.

Social workers are therefore necessarily involved in a constant dialogue – with themselves, with other agencies and professionals, with sponsoring bodies and with clients (or 'service users') about how far their work does (or should) promote care and/or control; independence and/or protection; dependency and/or empowerment. Social workers see the consequences of social disadvantage, which has led to a tradition of political action. A key component of this is a concern to recognise their position within social and political power structures and to ensure they do not reinforce discrimination and oppression, and challenge it where they can. This is reflected in commitment to the principles of anti-discriminatory and anti-oppressive practice (Dalrymple and Burke 2006, Dominelli 2002).

So, when thinking about social workers and interprofessional working it is important to bear in mind that their objectives are subject to constant debate and change according to wide social and political circumstances and the specific settings in which they are employed.

Social workers are expected to make difficult decisions not only when there is a balance of values to be struck but also when the outcomes of any decision cannot be clearly predicted. For example, they may help a frail older person who wishes to continue living in her own home to do so. Her rights to independence and self-determination may have been protected, but if she falls and is injured, in spite of all efforts to reduce the risk, it is all too easy to assume that this is the result of a bad decision.

Similarly, social workers recognise that it is generally better for children to be looked after in their own families, and are required to work in partnership with parents. So, unless there is clear evidence to the contrary, they will work to support a family to stay together during difficult times. However, it is often not possible to make a precise calculation of the extent of risk, and decisions about the right course of action are therefore complex. Social workers will be criticised for not having removed a child if a non-accidental injury occurs, but if they intervene too quickly too often, they will be criticised for highhandedness. A degree of professional wisdom is therefore called for and despite publicity to the contrary, social workers get things right more often than not (Ferguson 2002).

Social work organisation – history and current developments

Social work in the United Kingdom (UK) developed from at least four separate threads – charity, philanthropy, mutual aid and state intervention – that help to explain the existence of different perspectives about the nature and purpose of social work. Charity is part of Christian and other religious traditions. In the 19th century Christian charity was one of the explicit motivations for the visits of (most often) women of comfortable means who tried to alleviate poverty and improve morals. Philanthropy includes the efforts of late 19th and early 20th century reformers such as William Booth and Joseph Rowntree who undertook surveys of poverty and social deprivation. Traditions of mutual aid can be found in the friendly and cooperative societies and in the trade union movement. State intervention in welfare dates from the 19th century Poor Law which first gave us the concept of a deserving and a non-deserving poor; an idea that continues to influence social policy.

Social work in the UK developed after the Second World War with the creation of the welfare state, when local authority Welfare Departments were formed to work with older and disabled people and Children's Departments to work with children. The Local Authority Social Services Act 1970 (www.legislation.gov.uk) brought them together as single Social Services Departments. While social work has undergone many shifts in emphasis and organisational changes, the struggle to set up systems for effective interprofessional working has been a recurring theme for more than forty years.

The interprofessional dimension of social work with children and young people was developed organisationally by the New Labour government through the promotion of Children's Trusts. These brought together child care social work with schools, education departments and health services, alongside the development of services such as Sure Start (providing support to children and parents in the early years). However, Trusts were not developed by all local authorities, and more recently social work in this area has more commonly been provided in local authority agencies. A crucial development has been the requirement in the Children Act 2004 (www.legislation.gov.uk) for each authority to establish a Local Safeguarding Children Board that brings organisations together to agree on how they will safeguard and promote the welfare of children with an agreed set of local policies and procedures.

The interprofessional dimension of adult social work has been largely associated with the delivery of health and social care services. Some joint planning mechanisms were established as early as 1973 in the NHS Reorganisation Act (www.legislation.gov.uk). However, the New Labour government's promise to break down the 'Berlin Wall' between health and social services (DH 1998: 6.5) heralded a raft of policy and legislation aimed at bringing health and social care closer together. Obstacles to effective integration have included cultural differences between social workers and health professionals, but have often been as practical as incompatible funding arrangements or computer systems that cannot share information. In spite of these setbacks, however, there are an increasing number of examples of effective interprofessional teams which include social workers.

Qualification, registration and accountability

The Care Standards Act 2000 (www.legislation.gov.uk) provided the first legal protection for the title of social worker, only someone with a recognised qualification and registered is legally entitled to call themselves a social worker.

Between 2001 and 2012 social work was regulated by the General Social Care Council (GSCC) which set basic standards for social work education and practice. The Health and Social Care Act 2012 (www.legislation.gov.uk) abolished the GSCC and many of its functions were transferred to the Health and Care Professions Council (HCPC). Since 2003 the basic qualification for social work has been the completion of a three-year degree which replaced a two-year diploma.

Following the death of baby Peter Connelly in 2007 a series of reforms for social work education and practice were set out by the Social Work Task Force (DCSF 2009). A College of Social Work has been formed to represent the profession and promote standards of practice. A key element of these is the Professional Capabilities Framework (www.csw.org.uk) which is intended to set out standards for what social workers should know and be able to do when they qualify and as they develop once qualified.

Social work with children

Social work with children is principally governed by the 1989 and 2004 Children Acts (www.legislation.gov.uk) and associated legislation and guidance. One of the key ideas which informed the 1989 Act was the view that 'the child is a person and not an object of concern' (Butler-Sloss 1987: 254). The Act recognises the relationship between parents and children in terms of responsibility rather than rights. The legal frameworks emphasise the strengths and advantages of family life, based on evidence that arranging for children to be cared for away from their families cannot be presumed to make things better and might make them worse (DH 1991).

The 1989 Act places a duty on local authorities to promote the welfare of children in need and as far as possible to promote their upbringing in their own family. It also sets out criteria for deciding which children are in need and imposes duties on the local authority. Social workers assess the needs of specific children who have been identified as possibly being in need taking into account the children's individual development and characteristics, the ability of their parents to care for them, and their social circumstances. To look at these different aspects the Assessment Triangle assessment tool may be used (see Quinney, Thomas and Whittington 2009). In the spirit of the Children Acts 1989 and 2004 social workers seek to work in partnership with parents and children and other professionals to try to find constructive and cooperative solutions to what are often serious and long-standing difficulties. However, if a child is believed to be at risk of significant harm local authorities can seek legal powers to intervene through a supervision or care order.

Since Laming's (2003) report into the death of Victoria Climbié and the Children Act 2004 which followed, key policy and practice guidance has also been provided by *Every Child Matters* (Treasury 2003) and *Working Together to Safeguard Children* (DfE 2013). *Every Child Matters* aims to help every child fulfil their potential, and to move services away from a focus on whether a child is being abused or meets the thresholds for services.

▓ How might different professionals work together to help children fulfil their potential?

Social work with adults

The NHS and Community Care Act 1990 (NHSCCA) (www.legislation.gov. uk) represented a significant change in the way social work with adults is carried out in the UK. It remains the legal basis for the assessment of adults in need of social care services, although a range of other statutes govern the actual provision of services. Under the Act, responsibilities are placed on local authorities to coordinate and manage multiprofessional assessments of need and set-up of 'packages' of care. A typical care package coordinated by a social worker might combine free health care with means-tested services provided by the local authority or purchased by them from voluntary or private sector agencies. The Act requires social workers and health professionals to work closely together. While in most cases this improved the quality of the service provided, it also created enduring challenges for professionals seeking to combine a service that was free at the point of delivery (health) with a system involving strict eligibility criteria and thorough means testing (social care).

Since the 1990s, successive governments have promoted a policy agenda that has placed a growing emphasis on choice, independence and service user control. Direct payments to enable people in need of social care services to purchase and manage their own care were introduced in 1997 and extended a few years later. This was seen as a significant victory for disability rights campaigners and reflected a wider policy trend towards choice and consumer rights.

Subsequent policy documents mapped out Labour's and more recently the Coalition government's aspiration for a more 'personalised' approach to social care (DH 2012). Central to this policy is the concept of 'self directed support' whereby service users and carers have a high degree of control over how the money allocated to meet their assessed needs should be spent. This commonly takes the form of a 'personal budget' which can be paid directly to the service user or a trusted third party as a Direct Payment or can be administered by the local authority or a combination of the two.

An important dimension of the personalisation agenda is the concept of 'positive risk taking'. Nevertheless, growing numbers of very frail older people and an increasing awareness of the potential for exploitation and abuse of vulnerable people mean that the safeguarding and protection of vulnerable adults has become a key aspect of adult social work. Local authorities have the lead role in investigating suspected abuse or other safeguarding issues and in coordinating a multiagency safeguarding plan (DH 2000). The safeguarding of vulnerable adults is therefore an important focus for interprofessional working and often involves social workers working with the police as well as health professionals and care staff to keep people safe.

━━━━━━━━━━━━━━━ **ACTIVITY** ━━━━━━━━━━━━━━━

Look at the *No Secrets* guidance (DH 2000) and think about how you would work with the person involved and with other professionals if you were concerned about the safety of someone you were working with. If you work predominantly with children remember that you still would have a duty to raise concerns if you thought an adult was being abused.

Social workers need to understand the people they work with – their difficulties, strengths, but also the relationships they have with friends, family and others. Everything a social worker does must take place within legal and policy frameworks that determine their statutory responsibilities and the resources available to help as illustrated in the case study that follows.

CASE STUDY: The Williams Family

The family live on a housing estate in southern England. They moved from northern England two years ago to live near Mr Williams' elderly parents. Eric Williams is 43, and identifies himself as White. Jean Williams is 39 and identifies herself as Black. They have two children, Dan (13) and Mark (10).

Social workers first become involved when Dan's school contact the local education welfare service. Dan is often late for school in the morning and after lunch. In class, he seems to find concentration difficult and gets involved in fights. The school have contacted Mr and Mrs Williams who, although concerned, have been unable to meet with the teachers. Holly, an education welfare officer (and a qualified social worker), visits the home and talks first to the whole family, then to Mr and Mrs Williams together and to Dan and Mark individually. From these conversations Holly starts to develop a sense of the situation and how each member of the family sees it.

Eric Williams

Six months after the family moved Eric had a stroke. He followed a physical rehabilitation programme in hospital but has difficulty supporting his own weight and has limited mobility. Before he was discharged he was provided with some mobility aids (including a wheelchair), and some adaptations were made to the house. He also received advice about disability benefits. At home he needs help with washing and dressing and has difficulty managing many aspects of life that he used to take for granted.

No personal care services were arranged, as Eric believed he would be able to manage. However, he depends heavily on his eldest son as well as his wife for physical help. Mr Williams used to be a builder and ran a local football team. He now has little to occupy his time so watches a lot of television, reads the papers and plays computer games with his younger son in the evenings. He feels frustrated and depressed because he knows Jean is worried about their situation.

Jean Williams

Since her husband's stroke Jean has increased her hours working part-time in the local library and is now the main earner and worries as the mortgage repayments are hard to meet. She tries keeping these worries to herself and is seeking full-time work despite being unsure how she will find the time.

Jean is also concerned about Mark who, she thinks, is becoming cheeky and uncooperative. She was upset when local police suggested Mark might be involved in incidents of stealing from local shops. She says she has punished Mark by locking him in his room because she was so angry she might hit him.

Dan

Dan says he is late for school because he helps his father wash and dress and sometimes comes home to make his lunch. Dan wants to help his father and prefers this to life at school which is 'boring'. He misses going to football matches with his father and to the local football club he ran. When Holly asks what things he would most like to change he says 'to go out and do the things with friends that I used to do'. Dan knows his mother has been worried since his father's stroke. She seems too busy to spend time with him or his brother. Dan tries to steer clear when she gets angry and shouts at Mark.

Mr and Mrs Williams tell Holly that Dan is the only black child in his class. He has recently grown quickly and his classmates tease him about his clumsiness. They acknowledge that they have not been as involved with Dan's activities or schoolwork as they were before they moved.

Mark

Mark seems happy and easygoing. He appears to accept his father's situation and says he enjoys playing computer games with him. He agrees that recently his mother has often been angry with him and confirms that he is sometimes shut in his room when this happens. He denies stealing. When Holly asks what things he would most like to change he says that he wishes his mum would stop shouting at him.

Outcome of initial intervention

During this first contact, Holly demonstrated sensitivity and skill, earning a degree of trust from the family that has helped her assessment. Although Dan was the reason for Holly's involvement, he is plainly not the only person experiencing difficulties. He does need to improve his school attendance, but that is not the issue most on his mind. Of the two boys, Mark's situation is of greatest concern. Holly does not think that he is in immediate need of protection although he may be at risk of getting into trouble with the law or of being mistreated at home.

The indications are that Mr and Mrs Williams care a great deal about both children but are exhausted. Eric's stroke has had a significant impact on the family and there is an urgent need to consider how he and they might be helped to manage.

Discussing these findings with the family Holly tells them that, although there are ways in which she can help, she will also need to work with other professionals. They all agree she can talk to the teachers, contact the local child care team and the local adult community care team. Holly contacts the child care team to tell them that both Mark and Dan could be considered children in need and asks for their initial assessment. She asks the adult community care team for an assessment of Mr Williams' needs and tells both agencies of her referral to the other and of the plan to contact the schools.

The child care and adult care social workers

Managers in the two services see that there is the potential that the family, who have already talked to the education welfare officer, might now be visited separately by each service and asked for the same information. The family are already stressed and it is important not to make this worse. They discuss this and agree that their staff should work together and, initially, visit together. They also arrange for the child care social worker to be a black man and the adult care social worker a white woman. Although they do not know how much this matters to the family, they think this may help them develop trust and confidence in the service (Dominelli 1988).

The child care social worker, Darren, and the adult care social worker, Holly, have specific legal responsibilities (for more detail of the legislation see www.gov.uk):

■ under s. 17 of the Children Act 1989 – an assessment of children in need;
■ under s. 47 of the NHSCCA 1990 – an assessment of Mr Williams' need for community care services – and whether the local authority should provide services to meet them;
■ under the Carers (Recognition and Services) Act (1995) and The Carers and Disabled Children Act (2000) to assess Mrs Williams', Dan's, and possibly Mark's, needs as carers (Dan may feel he wants to help care for his father, and while this should not interfere with his education, it would be easy to overlook this aspect of his needs).

Initial visit

Meeting with the family shows that Darren and Holly understand that while their responsibilities are to ensure the well-being of the two boys on the one hand and Eric and his carers on the other, they are better addressed together. Though the two workers may need to make separate visits later, this first joint visit helps the family see these pieces of work as a whole.

Talking about their difficulties with the two social workers helps the family to see more clearly how they have been working hard to keep things going, and that they have been a great help to each other. They also see that it is time to talk more openly about the changes that have affected them and what changes they may now need to make.

Following this meeting, the workers visit again separately to complete their assessments.

Community care assessment

Holly asks Eric to complete a 'self assessment' questionnaire in order to identify the areas that concern him most, including the things that he would like to be able to do that are not possible at the moment. As the representative of the local authority Holly is responsible for assessing his needs under the NHSCCA. In doing so, she works with a physiotherapist and a community nurse who know Eric well and ensures that his own experience of his needs is at the centre of her assessment. Holly also undertakes a financial assessment in order to work out how much Eric will be asked to contribute to the cost of any support he receives. Once the assessment is completed, Holly is able to calculate an amount of money that is likely to be available to Eric as a personal budget to pay for the support he needs.

■ Why do you think it is important to involve the community nurse and physiotherapist in the assessment? What might be the advantages and disadvantages?

CASE STUDY continued

As well as working with Eric individually, Holly ensures that she considers the individual and interrelated needs of the whole family. This includes undertaking carer's assessments with Jean, Dan and Mark, with the possibility that one or more of them may be entitled to a carer's personal budget to help fund a break from the caring role.

Eric completes a support plan in discussion with his family and with help from Holly. The support plan outlines how Eric will spend his personal budget in order to meet his identified needs. He and Jean decide to take the personal budget as a direct payment so that Eric can arrange and pay for his support himself.

Eric uses his personal budget to employ a support worker to assist him with bathing and to help him get to the local pub. Holly finds out about a computer class at the local library which Eric enrols in and the physiotherapist arranges a short course of hydrotherapy with the aim of improving Eric's mobility and increasing his independence.

Children in need assessment

As part of the children in need assessment Darren contacts Holly about her discussions with the schools and speaks to a member of the local Youth Offending Team about the police reports.

Mark

Mark appears to have settled at his junior school. His teacher is pleased with his progress but observes that he is in a group of boys who can be very lively in school and sometimes get into trouble. She remembers a couple of occasions when Mark has been caught misbehaving and blamed for something which has involved others in the group. She wonders if Mark has been the scapegoat in the shoplifting incident as well.

Dan

Dan's teachers remain concerned about his attendance and performance at school. However, in the course of the assessment he talks to his mother about some bullying at school. Comments from other children have not just been teasing about clumsiness, but taunts about his ethnicity, and his dad's disability. She and Holly discuss this with his teachers, who investigate further and later confirm the bullying.

Planning meeting

Holly and Darren decide there is so much happening that it would help everyone to meet and coordinate plans. This meeting brings together Mr and Mrs Williams, the boys' teachers, a Youth Offending Team representative, Holly and Darren. It is chaired by a team manager. Dan and Mark decide not to attend but their views are represented at the meeting by a children's advocate who helped them write down their views on what should happen.

- What advantages can you see in bringing together the different professionals?
- What might be the tensions?
- Is there anyone not attending the meeting who would might need to know about any plans or outcomes? How might this information be passed on?

CASE STUDY continued

The proposed solutions
Dan's sports teacher offers to encourage him to talk to some other boys about joining a local under-14s football club. Dan is also told about the Young Carers project in the city but decides he would prefer to join the football club.

Dan's school decide to address the issue of potential racism within the school by making it the focus of a whole school project. Mark's school suggests he enrols in their after-school club. It is hoped this will give him time away from some of his peer group and allow Mrs Williams to make plans for full-time employment. The youth justice worker notes that Mark may have been unfairly associated with stealing and agrees to discuss this with the police. Darren undertakes to liaise with the other professionals involved and to meet the family again with Holly in a few weeks to discuss how the plans are working. This will give everyone a chance to review the solutions that have been put in place and agree any changes that might be needed.

Conclusion: the contribution of social work to interprofessional working

Social workers often have a key role in situations of the kind outlined in the case study, based on a social perspective that seeks to take into account how different aspects of a person's, or a family's, life work together to help them flourish or oppress or overwhelm them. Although it is not the only profession to draw on this perspective, social work tends to focus on enhancing and developing the networks within which people live, while a more individualised focus may appropriately be taken by other professions.

Social workers are increasingly likely to find themselves working alongside other health and social care professionals in unified interprofessional teams where they will often be legally charged with responsibility for coordinating interprofessional assessments. At their best the communication, networking and other social skills offered by social workers can make an invaluable contribution to team working and ensure that everyone involved works together in the most effective way.

RECOMMENDED READING

■ Quinney A. and Hafford-Letchfield T. (2012) *Interprofessional Social Work: Effective Collaborative Approaches.* London: Sage.

■ Whittington C., Thomas J. and Quinney A. (2009) *Interprofessional and Inter Agency Collaboration.* eLearning resource. www.scie.org.uk. Accessed February 2013.

■ Wilson K., Ruch G., Lymbery M. and Cooper A. (2011) *Social Work: An Introduction to Contemporary Practice.* London: Pearson Longman.

References

Adams R., Dominelli L. and Payne M. (eds) (2009) *Social Work: Themes, Issues and Critical Debates* (3rd edn). Basingstoke: Palgrave.

Butler-Sloss E. (1987) *Report of the Inquiry into Child Abuse in Cleveland 1987.* London: DHSS.

Coulshed V. and Orme J. (1998) *Social Work Practice.* Basingstoke: Macmillan.

(CSW) College of Social Work (2009) *The Contribution of Social Work.* London TCSW. www.tcsw.org.uk. Accessed June 2013.

Dalrymple J. and Burke B. (2006) *Anti-Oppressive Practice: Social Care and the Law* (2nd edn). Buckingham: Open University Press.

DCSF (Department for Children Schools and Families) (2009) *Building a Safe, Confident Future – The Final Report of the Social Work Task Force.* London: The Stationery Office.

DfE (Department for Education) (2013) *Working together to Safeguard Childern.* www.education. gov.uk. Accessed January 2014.

DH (Department of Health) (1991) *Patterns and Outcomes in Child Placement.* London: HMSO.

DH (1998) *Modernising Social Services: Promoting Independence, Improving Protection, Raising Standards.* CM 4169. London: The Stationery Office.

DH (2000) *No Secrets: Guidance on Developing and Implementing Multi-agency Policies and Procedures to Protect Vulnerable Adults from Abuse.* London: DH.

DH (2012) *Caring for our Future: Reforming Care and Support.* London: The Stationery Office.

Dominelli L. (1988) *Anti-Racist Social Work.* Basingstoke: Macmillan.

Dominelli L. (2002) Values in social work: contested entities with enduring qualities. In Adams R., Dominelli L. and Payne M. (eds), *Critical Practice in Social Work.* Basingstoke: Palgrave, pp. 15–27.

Ferguson H. (2002) Blame culture in child protection. *The Guardian,* 16th January.

IASSW/IFSW (International Association of Schools of Social Work/International Federation of Social Workers) (2001) www.iassw-aiets.org. Accessed December 2012.

Laming, Lord (2003) *The Victoria Climbié Inquiry: Report of an Inquiry* Cm 5730. London: The Stationery Office.

Quinney A., Thomas J. and Whittington C. (2009) *Working Together to Assess Needs, Strengths and Risks.* elearning resource. www.scie.org.uk. Accessed February 2013.

Treasury (2003) *Every Child Matters Cm 5860.* Chief Secretary to the Treasury. London: The Stationery Office.

Trevithick P. (2012) *Social Work Skills: A Practice Handbook* (3rd edn). Buckingham: Open University Press.

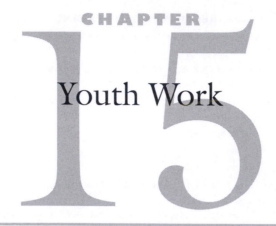

CHAPTER 15

Youth Work

Billie Oliver and Bob Pitt

Introduction

This chapter presents the aims and purpose of youth work: what it is, where it happens and who does it. It outlines the roles of youth workers and how they work, illustrated with case studies from practice. It offers a flavour of debates and issues facing youth work as a result of the opportunities and tensions created by recent transformations of these services. Opportunities include the integration of services and the challenge of collaborative working with different professionals for the benefit of young people.

What is youth work?

Young (1999) argues that youth work's purpose lies in enabling and supporting young peoples' capacity to take charge of their lives and to participate in decision-making processes in their community. Youth work is about 'exploring values' (Young 1999: 4): a purpose distinct from inculcating particular values in young people; it is not an activity of imposition, its intention is 'to liberate as opposed to domesticate' (Young 1999: 79). Youth work involves adults accepting, valuing and building relationships with young people based on 'honesty, trust, respect and reciprocity' (Young 1999: 5). The challenge for practitioners is to explain 'in contemporary language, how and why this is done' (Williamson 2005: 81).

Youth workers work with young people aged 11–25, although those who make most use of the service tend to be aged 13–19 (NYA 2012). At its core the aim of youth work is to support personal and social development. Its distinctive characteristics include the voluntary and active involvement of young people in developing provision of informal educational opportunities as the primary method of engagement.

> Youth work helps young people learn about themselves, others and society through non-formal educational activities that combine enjoyment, challenge, learning and achievement.
>
> (NYA 2012)

The youth work sector consists of local authority, voluntary/community and national providers including uniformed, sports and faith-based organisations. Smith (2002) notes that the variety of perspectives of what counts as youth work requires a recognition that there are different forms of youth work rather than a single practice. Youth work may appear as 'an ambiguous set of practices, pushed in different directions at different times by different interests' (Bradford 2005: 58) yet underlying its different guises is the commitment to 'voluntary ... [and] participatory' (Bradford 2005: 58) relationships with young people.

QUESTIONS

- Why is the voluntary participation of young people in engagement with services and youth workers important?
- How might participation in youth work activities help build confidence and self-esteem?

The voluntary nature of activity for young people of choosing to use services contrasts with the statutory duties of other professionals such as social workers, who may be obligated to intervene in the lives of families or individuals. Youth work encourages and supports young people, gives them responsibility, encourages participation, and helps build confidence and self-esteem during the transition from dependence to independence. Youth work enables young people to become involved with their communities as active citizens in national and local programmes or schemes such as the National Citizen Service and Duke of Edinburgh's Award.

Youth work is built on establishing trust with groups or individuals, requiring youth workers to be non-judgemental and make use of conversation, chat and activities to engage with young people. The aim is to draw young people towards informal educational opportunities to explore issues that affect their lives, such as sexual health, drug and alcohol misuse, bullying, sexism and racism. Youth work offers both spontaneous and planned opportunities for young people to learn about themselves, others and wider society. Good youth work is 'well prepared and highly disciplined, yet improvised' (Davies 2010: 6).

Historical and policy context

Youth work has experienced fluctuations in popularity and struggled to gain governmental recognition as a profession. The Albermarle Committee was established in 1958 to review the Youth Service in response to concerns related to: increasing numbers of young people; the ending of National Service; rising youth crime; and the perceived reduction in deference shown by young people towards their elders amid an emerging youth culture born of increasing affluence (ME 1960).

Later reports such as *Learning to Succeed* (DfEE 1999) and *Bridging the Gap* (SEU 1999) identified risks for young people when agencies and professionals work in isolation without effective communication. The government introduced the Connexions Service (DfEE 2000) to provide holistic support and to prevent vulnerable young people from 'falling through the net' of the various services. The core of the analysis viewed the ineffectiveness of youth provision as caused by the proliferation of specialist agencies dealing with disconnected parts of the young person's life: 'young people often feel as if they are being passed from pillar to post and each time they meet an official from yet another agency they have to tell their story again' (Merton 1998: 21).

Transforming Youth Work (DfEE 2001) followed a series of OFSTED reports criticising the quality of some local authority youth services, noting variations in funding between authorities, and acknowledging difficulties in recruiting, training and retaining youth workers. Together with the Connexions Service, *Transforming Youth Work* moved youth work away from its core values towards a more individualised, outcome-focused and target-driven model seeking to prioritise young people's participation in education, employment and citizenship. For Smith (2000), the introduction of the Connexions Strategy was 'deeply problematic' as it entailed a 'considerable narrowing of focus'. In other UK nation states, innovation rather than imitation can be identified in, for example, the Wales policy document *Extending Entitlement* (NAW 2000).

Laming (2003) concluded that children's needs were neglected by a failure of joined-up working, poor information sharing systems, and an over-reliance on professional and agency boundaries. In response, *Every Child Matters* (DfES 2003) called for the creation of services and working practices emphasising service integration through multiagency working and partnerships between the voluntary, community and statutory sectors. *Every Child Matters* led to the Children Act 2004 (www.legislation.gov.uk) and to local authority-based integrated children and young people's services with a key strategic aim of enabling cross-professional boundary work with children and young people. A further report, *Youth Matters* (DfES 2005a), proposed a single, integrated youth support service within local authorities. These policy responses amounted to restructuring of services and shifting responsibilities for who did what, where and with whom.

Aiming High for Young People set out a ten-year strategy to help young people in England, particularly those in deprived areas, participate in enjoyable and 'purposeful activities' (DCSF 2007: 22) in their free time to develop new skills and raise their aspirations. In Wales, *Young People, Youth Work, Youth Services* set out a national strategy based on entitlements for every young person aged 11 to 25 ensuring opportunities to engage in 'meaningful activities that are challenging, creative and exciting ... [and] to participate in the planning, design, management and evaluation of all provision' (NAW 2007: 13). The Scottish government produced *Moving Forward: A Strategy for Improving Young People's Chances through Youth Work* (SE 2007).

In response to *Positive for Youth* (DfE 2011a) many local authorities have found innovative and collaborative ways to offer integrated youth support services in new youth centre hubs. *Positive for Youth* sets out the Coalition government's view of the contribution of youth workers:

Youth workers …can offer young people high quality opportunities for informal learning … help young people develop the strong aspirations they need to realise their potential … listen to young people, and build their confidence and skill to make their voice heard in decisions.

(DfE 2011a: 15)

Policy trends reflect government thinking about young people and the purposes of youth work, addressing concerns ranging from 'moral panic' (Cohen 1972) regarding the behaviour of young people to the need to secure youth service provision during a period of public spending cuts. Along the way government has sought to connect specialist agencies, tackle youth unemployment, safeguard children and young people through interprofessional working, raise aspirations and promote active citizenship.

Where does youth work take place?

Along with the importance placed on autonomy, Williamson (1997) emphasised young people's desire for safe spaces to meet, make decisions, get advice and talk to people other than parents or friends. Local authorities, voluntary organisations and independent groups offer youth services. Youth work takes place wherever young people meet although it traditionally occurs as *centre-based work* in youth clubs or community centres. *Detached youth work* happens on the street where youth workers attempt to contact young people who do not use centres. Youth work also takes place in schools or colleges during lunch or after school, or as classroom contributions to personal, social and health education, and the citizenship curriculum. As *outreach work*, youth workers develop provision with and for young people. It might involve setting up specialist projects aimed at particular groups, such as young people in danger of exclusion from school, or dealing with issues like drug misuse; and mobile projects where, for example, a converted bus takes workers and resources to communities.

CASE STUDY: a youth drop-in centre

The centre is situated in a small town operating to appeal to all young people, with a priority target group of 13- to 19-year-olds. The local authority pays the running costs and employs a manager and part-time staff offering day and evening drop-in sessions. The centre has a pool table, television lounge, computers with free Internet access and a coffee bar run by the young people. The centre operates as an informal space for young people to chat and chill.

The lunchtime sessions attract young people from the local school or those without a job; those who have fallen out of the school system or dropped out of college; and former regulars, such as young mums. Lunchtime sessions tend towards an even gender mix and the young people stay for about an hour. They often have individual queries or issues where other agencies or services such as careers, housing, benefits and health and social services may be involved. One morning each week the local Careers Service provides an information session.

> The centre runs two sessions a week with pupils from the local secondary school. One focuses on a youth award scheme with a group of year 10 pupils; the other provides an alternative to school for a group of disengaged year 11 pupils. Over several weeks a programme emerged involving music production on computer, a singing performance, band practices, gaining youth award credits through cookery, producing CDs, and a pool tournament.
>
> The evening sessions attract predominantly males who tend to stay longer giving the centre manager a chance to help the young people negotiate their own programme of informal education. Typically this might involve watching a DVD on alcohol misuse followed by discussion, organising trips to tenpin bowling, planning a residential trip to an outdoor activity centre, decorating the television lounge, or devising a dance night competition.

As with other public services there has been a move towards multiagency partnership working. Youth services commonly work with other services including housing, youth justice, police, health, social services and education in order to meet the needs and aspirations of young people. This interagency work can make use of particular expertise, signpost specific services, and share good practice (Sapin 2009: 37). Within partnerships, youth workers may take on a variety of roles including advocate or mentor working with young people to gain access to services and to create opportunities.

QUESTIONS

- What challenges might there be for centre workers to meet the needs of different groups?
- In what situations might youth workers need to work with other professionals?

The professional role, accountability and boundaries in youth work

In 2005, the *Children's Workforce Strategy* (DfES 2005b) listed just five titles under the heading of 'Youth Work & related roles': youth worker, personal adviser, learning mentor, education welfare officer, and key worker. However, a Young People's Workforce in England report (CWDC 2009) identified youth work as one component of an increasingly complex and fragmented young people's workforce listing some of the new professional roles emerging such as: extended schools worker, family support advisor, play ranger, leaving care worker, substance use worker and youth support worker (Oliver and Pitt 2011: 139).

Tucker differentiates between 'youth working' and youth work suggesting that ways of working with young people tend to change over time in response to differing demands and priorities, with the result that an occupational identity for youth working 'has never been fixed' (2005: 212). The title *youth worker* does not have protected professional status meaning that youth work is not necessarily undertaken by professionally qualified people. However, new national occupational standards (Lifelong Learning UK 2012) provide a framework for the requirements of qualified youth workers. From 2010 a nationally qualified professional youth worker will have an honours (or higher) degree; and local qualifications are available for youth support workers. Local and national qualifications are validated and approved by the National Youth Agency.

Key skills for youth work include the ability to:

- Build relationships and engage with young people
- Engage in critical dialogue and work with young people in promoting their rights
- Promote young people's self awareness, confidence and participation
- Facilitate learning and development of young people through youth work
- Plan and implement learning activities in youth work
- Safeguard the health and welfare of young people
- Promote inclusion, equity and the valuing of diversity

(Lifelong Learning UK 2012: 6)

Youth workers aim to engage young people in a range of activities and to 'foster environments for learning' (Robertson 2005: 18), primarily through informal education and working with the concerns, activity or interests of individuals or groups. Informal educators start 'where people are, with their own preoccupations and in their own places' (Batsleer 2008: 5) and learning occurs because it is of 'immediate significance ... rather than derived from a pre-established curriculum' (Batsleer 2008: 5). Informal education does not have preconceived ideas concerning outcome, rather it is unpredictable and used as a methodology for building relationships that value respect and reciprocity.

Conversation is central to informal education; and to build and maintain trust with young people, workers must be 'fair, truthful, punctilious about fulfilling obligations, thoughtful and unselfish in their conduct' (Jeffs and Smith 2005: 98). For Smith (2005) the skill of informal education is to 'catch the moment' in conversations with people in order to 'deepen their thinking or to put themselves in touch with their feelings' with the aim of 'exploring or enlarging' their experience.

This 'professional friendship' (Greenop 2011: 49) approach can lead to a blurring of boundaries and accountabilities. Ledwith and Springett note the potential ethical dangers of influencing the views of those less powerful in this 'fragile process' (2010: 138) of trying to enter into equal conversations and dialogues with others. Batsleer warns against the danger of 'manipulation and brainwashing' (2008: 136) if youth workers are insufficiently reflective about the impact of their power and influence. She argues that what is needed is an 'understanding of the ethics of closeness' (2008: 105), and insight by practitioners into the importance of their role in creating a 'professional boundary for a safe space in which learning can occur' (2008: 105).

Ethical principles

Youth work is informed by a commitment to the principle of equality of opportunity. Key concepts in youth work are choice, freedom, responsibility and justice. Effective youth work offers young people opportunities to meet others from different racial, cultural and religious backgrounds and to support them to increase their understanding of others. Banks suggests that, like other professions, youth work embodies concerns about 'professional integrity, trustworthiness and honesty of its practitioners' (2010: 4) as they face challenges of balancing 'roles of carer, protector, advocate and liberator' (2010: 4) in striving to respect young people's rights and cultural diversity while working for participatory democracy.

Youth workers follow the statement of principles of ethical conduct established by the National Youth Agency with a commitment to:

- Treat young people with respect …
- Respect and promote young people's rights to make their own decisions and choices…
- Promote and ensure the welfare and safety of young people …
- Contribute towards the promotion of social justice …

Youth workers have a commitment to:

- Recognise the boundaries between personal and professional life …
- Recognise the need to be accountable …
- Develop and maintain the required skills and competence …
- Work for conditions in employing agencies where these principles are discussed, evaluated and upheld.

(NYA 2004: 6)

These ethical principles create dilemmas for youth workers in situations where betraying a confidence or undermining trust is required because of, for example, an issue of child protection or safety. A new code of ethics was drafted by the National Youth Agency in summer 2013. This was done in preparation for the launch of the Institute for Youth Work in England 'to promote quality youth work and secure standards for ethical, effective practice' (NYA 2013). The code covers issues such as protecting young people's privacy and ensuring youth workers do not have sexual relationships with young people (Lepper 2013). Membership of the new Institute will be open to professional, volunteer and student youth workers who will be required to sign up to the ethical code.

CASE STUDY continued

The drop-in centre manager, Yvonne, was asked by an education welfare officer from the local youth offending team to cooperate with a truancy sweep organised by the education welfare service, police and local school. Rather than use the police station or school, the education welfare officer wanted to use the centre as neutral territory to bring young people picked up in the sweep.

Yvonne was more interested in why young people truant rather than who or how many, and she thought that using the centre could undermine the commitment to honesty and to not 'grassing up' young people to the school authorities. After discussion with centre staff Yvonne believed that to maintain relationships of trust with the young people, it was fair to inform them that the centre would be used as part of a planned truancy sweep.

Yvonne explained the centre principles to the education welfare officer and asked when, where and why this sweep was happening; and what would happen to the young people picked up. They agreed that Yvonne would let those who attend the centre know the week, but not the day, of the sweep.

QUESTIONS

■ Do you think Yvonne's action appropriate? If so, why? If not, why not?

■ What are the potential advantages and disadvantages of using the centre in this way?

Under certain circumstances (such as in cases of child protection) statutory duties override confidentiality. However, the values and principles of 'empowerment, participation, collective welfare and social justice' and associated 'value-based activity' (Banks 2003: 104) can lead to misunderstandings or conflict with other professionals. The move towards Integrated Youth Support Services, introduced as part of the Connexions Service, has highlighted differences between professions and raised issues of accountability, confidentiality and professional boundaries. Tensions related to a perceived requirement to perform a policing role through surveillance and record keeping (Smith 2003) raise dilemmas for youth workers in regards to disclosing information without the consent of the young person.

Work with young people in communities requires interagency and interprofessional collaboration between different, organisations, interest groups and individuals with varying systems, cultures and values. Differences in professional cultures and values can lead to 'client dilemmas' (Lindsay 1995: 493) for practitioners between obligations towards young people and professional accountability and responsibility. In the case study above, the youth worker must choose between maintaining the trust and respect of the drop-in centre attendees on the one hand and, on the other, cooperating with the truancy sweep. This illustrates an inherent contradiction between the aspirations of youth work and constraints of compulsory school attendance.

CASE STUDY continued

Kate first ran away from home when she was 12: 'I didn't get on with my step-dad'. She walked around until after dark and was brought home by the police. She ran away next when she was 13 spending the night at a friend's house. 'No one cared. No one came looking for me.' The third time she was careful not to get caught by the police: 'I walked around all night by my mum's house. It was scary and cold.'

Rees (2011) estimates that 8.9 per cent of young people under 16 have run away for at least one night and that no fewer than 55 per cent of these have run away from home on more than one occasion. Running away increases the risk of entering care and adult homelessness. The main trigger for running away is family problems. Most runaways return home or are returned but many do not receive help with their problems.

The weekend Kate, age 14, spent sleeping in a bus shelter, she was returned home by the police who referred her to Mehri, a youth engagement worker in the neighbourhood locality team attached to Kate's school. They met at the local youth drop-in centre to explore Kate's concerns and identify her options.

Mehri, a qualified youth worker, had little experience of working with runaways so contacted a local voluntary agency specialising in helping young runaways. All parties agreed that, because of their existing relationship, Mehri would continue to work with Kate. Kate agreed to include her mother and stepfather in a meeting where they would each have the opportunity to talk about their experience of the situation. Mehri advocated for Kate when it appeared Kate's mother was not recognising points Kate was trying to make. They agreed on some strategies and boundaries to try to help Kate feel less excluded. For example, Kate's mother agreed to spend a specific amount of time with her daughter each week and Kate agreed to keep her mother informed of her whereabouts outside of the home.

During the next two months Kate and Mehri met weekly to assess Kate's situation in regard to her family. Kate has become comfortable and relaxed about going to the youth drop-in centre. She has engaged in group work and informal conversations about living at home and the dangers of running away. She has made new friends and feels she has a safe place to go, with people she can talk to.

Debates and issues in youth work

The public spending cuts of the Coalition government will impact local authority statutory youth work and services: North Somerset Council presented plans to cut the youth service budget by more than 70 per cent by 2014/15 (Puffett 2012) and South Gloucestershire council proposed targeted specialist services, outreach work and one-to-one support to replace youth clubs (Mahadevan 2012). The Coalition government expects a mix of voluntary-community sector and business to fill the gap stating 'the voluntary and community sector sits at the heart of the government's ambitions to create a Big Society' (DCLG 2010: 3).

The *Big Society* agenda is 'a call to action' where 'citizens, communities and civil society providers all need to play a part in reducing the deficit' (DCLG 2010: 12). At the launch of the *Positive for Youth* strategy the government envisioned local authorities building partnerships with voluntary organisations and businesses to lead 'the way with innovative projects that are inspiring young people' (DfE 2011b). The aims are to make savings while finding better ways of doing things. The debates here centre on who should provide services. By drawing in business the Coalition is interested in involving or establishing social enterprises: profit-making organisations operating with social purpose.

In Defence of Youth Work (IDYW 2009) campaigns to protect youth services in the UK. It is concerned with maintaining democratic and emancipatory forms of youth work 'to tip the balance of power in young people's favour' (Nicholls 2012: 40). *In Defence of Youth Work* is concerned not just about who provides youth work and services but what is provided and how. For example, the campaign emphasises 'the sanctity of the voluntary principle', 'a commitment to conversations' and 'the importance of association' (IDYW 2009).

Cuts in youth work and services can be seen in a wider context of nearly one million young people not in employment, education or training (Adonis 2012). It has been noted that 'the idea of integrated working in the children and youth workforce seems to be enjoying something of a renaissance at present' (Ennals 2011: 16). One way forward is to explore how professionals working with and for young people can work together to address three priorities highlighted by the Commission on Youth Unemployment that recognises young people need 'more job opportunities to be available here and now'; 'better preparation and motivation for work'; and 'support of a far more active welfare state' (Adonis 2012).

Conclusion: the future of youth work

Youth work in the UK 'occupies an ambivalent space' by appearing as both 'under threat' and 'being valued and in demand, on condition that it constantly reinvents itself' (Batsleer 2010: 153). One debate that followed the introduction of the Connexions Service centred on threats to the professional identity of youth workers. Tucker had previously identified the challenges to professional identity in youth working, defined as 'shorthand for the occupational activities involved in the fields of health, welfare and education' (2004: 81) before going on to note that 'youth working appears to be changing at a rapid rate' (2004: 82). There were fears that some youth work approaches would be lost with a shift of emphasis to formal rather than informal education and by targets set for the number of young people achieving accreditation for personal and social development. Youth workers, it was feared, could become mere employment and training brokers concerned with placing individuals in employment rather than with valuing the principles of voluntary associational activity (Smith 2003).

Debates continue about what counts as youth work and whether the voluntary relationship between youth worker and young person is important. Questions remain about whether youth work should provide a service for all young people, or should target particular groups, take on individual casework and shift towards formal education. Some argue that opportunities for young people to be involved in association, activities and autonomy are being lost due to the decline in traditional settings such as the youth club (Robertson 2005). Youth work, however, continues with a substantial amount of voluntary youth work independent of government funding and resources, being maintained and developed through uniformed, sports and faith-based organisations. Taking a wider view of what counts as youth work illustrates that young people are for the most part active members of their community achieving transition from child to adult alongside dedicated and well-trained paid and volunteer youth workers operating to clear, ethical and professional principles.

Over the last twenty years the socio-political climate for public sector professionals working with young people has changed so fundamentally that there is a need to understand not only the nature of that change but also how it impacts on the professional work and identities of particular individuals and groups. Interprofessional opportunities to link up and explore these issues come from 'a renewal of practitioner networks seeking to defend critical and radical professional practice' (Batsleer 2010: 164) in fields such as youth work and social work. While Jeffs and Smith note 'a certain despondency has infected state-sponsored youth work', they recognise 'a lot remains that is vibrant and healthy' (2010: 14). Their evidence derives from the narratives of practitioners describing how they and others 'carve out space to develop relationships, engage in conversation and build communities with young people' (2010: 14). Successful interprofessional working to benefit young people will result from youth workers gaining more confidence about what they have to offer in terms of their creative skills, professional knowledge and innovative practices, and actively seeking to share these with other professions.

RECOMMENDED READING

- Harrison R., Benjamin C., Curran S. and Hunter R. (eds) (2007) *Leading Work with Young People*. Milton Keynes: Open University Press/Sage.
- NYA (National Youth Agency) (2012) *Guide to Youth Work and Youth Services*. www.nya.org.uk. Accessed January 2013.
- Roberts J. (2009) *Youth Work Ethics*. Exeter: Learning Matters.
- Soni S. (2011) *Working with Diversity in Youth and Community Work*. Exeter: Learning Matters.

References

Adonis, Lord (2012) Debate on 'Youth Unemployment' House of Lords 14th June. www.publications.parliament.uk. Accessed January 2013.

Banks S. (2003) Conflicts of culture and accountability. In Banks S., Butcher H., Henderson P. and Robertson J. (eds), *Managing Community Practice: Principles, Policies and Programmes*. Bristol: Policy Press, pp. 103–20.

Banks S. (2010) Ethics and the youth worker. In Banks S. (ed.), *Ethical Issues in Youth Work* (2nd edn). Abingdon: Routledge, pp. 3–23.

Batsleer J.R. (2008) *Informal Learning in Youth Work*. London: Sage.

Batsleer J. (2010) Youth work prospects: back to the future? In Batsleer J. and Davies B. (eds), *What Is Youth Work?* Exeter: Learning Matters, pp. 153–65.

Bradford S. (2005) Modernising youth work: from the universal to the particular and back again. In Harrison R. and Wise C. (eds), *Working with Young People*. London: Sage, pp. 57–70.

Cohen S. (1972) *Folk Devils and Moral Panics*. London: MacGibbon and Kee.

CWDC (Children's Workforce Development Council) (2009) *A Picture Worth Millions: State of the Young People's Workforce*. Leeds: CWDC.

Davies B. (2010) What do we mean by youth work? In Batsleer J. and Davies B. (eds), *What Is Youth Work?* Exeter: Learning Matters, pp. 1–6.

DCLG (Department for Communities and Local Government) (2010) *Building a Stronger Civil Society*. London: DCLG.

DCSF (Department for Children, Schools and Families) (2007) *Aiming High for Young People: A Ten Year Strategy for Positive Activities*. London: HM Treasury.

DfE (Department for Education) (2011a) *Positive for Youth: A New Approach to Cross-Government Policy for Young People aged 13 to 19*. London: HM Government.

DfE (2011b) Government sets out strategy to be Positive for Youth. Press notice. 19th December, updated 26th April 2012.

DfEE (Department for Education and Employment) (1999) *Learning to Succeed: A New Framework for Post-16 Learning.* London: The Stationery Office.

DfEE (2000) *The Connexions Service: Prospectus and Specification.* Nottingham: DfEE.

DfEE (2001) *Transforming Youth Work: Developing Youth Work for Young People.* Nottingham: DfEE.

DfES (Department for Education and Skills) (2003) *Every Child Matters.* Nottingham: DfES.

DfES (2005a) *Youth Matters.* Cm 6629. Nottingham: DfES.

DfES (2005b) *The Children's Workforce Strategy: A Strategy to Build a World-Class Workforce for Children and Young People.* Nottingham: DfES.

Ennals P. (2011) Integrated working makes a comeback. *Children and Young People Now.* 1st–14th November.

Greenop D. (2011) Mentoring: a qualitative evaluation of what works and what does not. *Youth and Policy* 107: 34–54.

IDYW (In Defence of Youth Work) (2009) *The Open Letter.* www.indefenceofyouthwork.org.uk. Accessed January 2013.

Jeffs T. and Smith M.K. (2005) *Informal Education: Conversation, Democracy and Learning* (3rd edn). Nottingham: Educational Heretics.

Jeffs T. and Smith M.K. (2010) Introducing youth work. In Jeffs T. and Smith M.K. (eds), *Youth Work Practice.* Basingstoke: Palgrave Macmillan, pp. 1–14.

Laming, Lord (2003) *Inquiry into the Death of Victoria Climbié.* London: TSO.

Ledwith M. and Springett J. (2010) *Participatory Practice: Community Based Action for Transformative Change.* Bristol: Policy Press.

Lepper J. (2013) Youth work institute unveils draft code of ethics. *Children and Young People Now.* 1st July.

Lifelong Learning UK (2012) *National Occupational Standards for Youth Work.* www.nya.org.uk. Accessed January 2013.

Lindsay G. (1995) Values, ethics and psychology. *The Psychologist.* **8**: 493–8.

Mahadevan J. (2012) Council plans youth club and children's centre closures, *CYP Now.* 13th April.

Merton B. (1998) *Finding the Missing.* Leicester: Youth Work Press.

ME (Ministry of Education) (1960) *The Youth Service in England and Wales ('The Albemarle Report').* London: Her Majesty's Stationery Office, Chapter 1.

NAW (National Assembly for Wales) (2000) *Extending Entitlement: Supporting Young People in Wales.* Report by Policy Unit, National Assembly for Wales, September.

NAW (2007) *Young People, Youth Work, Youth Services: National Youth Service Strategy for Wales.* NAW.

Nicholls D. (2012) *For Youth Workers and Youth Work.* Bristol: Policy Press.

NYA (National Youth Agency) (2004) *Ethical Conduct in Youth Work: A Statement of Values and Principles.* Leicester: NYA.

NYA (2012) *About NYA.* www.nya.org.uk. Accessed January 2013.

NYA (2013) *Institute for Youth Work: Background.* www.nya.org.uk. Accessed July 2013.

Oliver B. and Pitt B. (2011) The children's workforce: new roles and career opportunities. In Oliver B. and Pitt B. (eds), *Working with Children, Young People and Families.* Exeter: Learning Matters, pp. 137–51.

Puffett N. (2012) Young person launches legal challenge against youth cuts. *Children and Young People Now.* 25th April.

Rees G. (2011) *Still Running 3: Early Findings from our Third National Survey of Young Runaways.* London: Children's Society.

Robertson S. (2005) *Youth Clubs: Association, Participation, Friendship and Fun!* Lyme Regis: Russell House.

Sapin K. (2009) *Essential Skills for Youth Work Practice*. London: Sage.

SE (Scottish Executive) (2007) *Moving Forward: A Strategy for Improving Young People's Chances through Youth Work*. Edinburgh: Scottish Executive.

SEU (Social Exclusion Unit) (1999) *Bridging the Gap,* Cm 4405. London: SEU/TSO.

Smith M.K. (2000) The Connexions Service in England. *The Encyclopaedia of Informal Education*. www.infed.org. Last update 29th May 2012. Accessed January 2013.

Smith M.K. (2002) Youth work: an introduction. *The Encyclopaedia of Informal Education*. www.infed.org. Accessed January 2013.

Smith M.K. (2003) The end of youth work? *Young People Now*. 5th–11th February.

Smith M.K. (2005) Introducing informal education. *The Encyclopaedia of Informal Education*. www.infed.org. Accessed January 2013.

Tucker S. (2004) Youth working: professional identities given, received or contested. In Roche J., Tucker S., Thompson R. and Flynn R. (eds), *Youth in Society*. London: Sage, pp. 81–9.

Tucker S. (2005) The sum of the parts – exploring youth working identities. In Harrison R. and Wise C. (eds), *Working with Young People*. London: Sage, pp. 204–13.

Williamson H. (1997) *Youth and Policy: Contexts and Consequences*. Aldershot: Ashgate.

Williamson H. (2005) Challenging practice: a personal view on youth work in times of changed expectations. In Harrison R. and Wise C. (eds), *Working with Young People*. London: Sage/Open University, pp. 70–85.

Young K (1999). *The Art of Youth Work*. Lyme Regis: Russell House.

The Future for Interprofessional Working

16

New and Emerging Roles

Judith Thomas, Gary Smart and Kevin Stone

Introduction

This chapter explores some of the ways that traditional role boundaries are changing and how this impacts on service delivery. To illustrate some of the challenges that change creates we focus on two contrasting roles – that of the *approved mental health practitioner* and the *specialist paramedic* – to illustrate the way in which roles are changing and expanding as in the case of the latter and, in relation to the former, how a role previously undertaken by one professional can now be undertaken by a much wider range of professionals. The chapter is written by professionals and academics who have witnessed and are now involved in the resulting changes to service delivery. The first section is written by GS, a specialist paramedic who is involved in educating these professionals for their expanding role. The second section is written by KS, a social worker who is now an approved mental health practitioner and JT, also a social worker who used to specialise in mental health work and more recently has been involved in teaching and researching interprofessional learning and working.

Specialist paramedic

The ambulance service is a critical component of the urgent and emergency healthcare system in the United Kingdom (UK). Ambulance personnel deal daily with an extraordinary range and severity of conditions, ranging from mild fevers to massive multiple traumas. The work they do is challenging, emotional, at times dangerous, and often highly rewarding. The ambulance service response encompasses the primary stages of the emergency care pathway including responding to emergency 999 calls; dispatch of personnel to the scene of an illness or trauma; and triage, treatment and transport by ambulance or air-ambulance. In 2009–10, 8.2 million emergency 999 calls were responded to by ambulance crews across England and Wales (NAO 2011, WAS 2011). The speed of response and quality of care are critical factors to the ultimate outcome (Bradley 2005, NAO 2011). The service is increasingly recognised as having a wider role, as a gateway to other NHS services and ensuring that service users can access the care they need close to their home (NAO 2011).

The role of the specialist paramedic, sometimes referred to as the *emergency care practitioner*, is an initiative focused on utilising the existing knowledge and experience of emergency healthcare professionals and expanding their expertise and scope of practice (MA 2004). At the time of writing, there is some confusion of titles for this role; 'specialist paramedic' is the term used in the NHS Allied Health Professions Career Framework and is considered the correct description by their professional body, the College of Paramedics, as it provides greater clarity for the public as to which profession is providing treatment (Bradley 2011). Specialist paramedic is also preferred by the UK statutory regulator, the Health and Care Professions Council (HCPC), as it uses a designation containing the legally protected professional title.

The specialist paramedic (SPM) role builds upon the primary role of the paramedic who is the registered healthcare professional and senior clinician on an ambulance. Paramedics are educated to degree or diploma level undertaking placements as part of their training primarily with the ambulance service; but to foster greater interprofessional understanding placements also include areas such as Emergency Departments (EDs), children's EDs, operating departments and central delivery suites. The White Paper *Taking Healthcare to the Patient* (Bradley 2005) recommended that paramedic education should have greater commonality with other health professionals within higher education, rather than the ambulance service providing the training. It also recommended that their career pathways should be integrated within the wider NHS, so in addition to their primary qualification, SPMs must complete an additional degree level programme with a minimum of 400 hours designated theory learning and 1,000 hours learning in appropriate placements such as Minor Injury Units, NHS Walk-in-Centres and Primary Care locations (SFH 2007). Large proportions of existing educational programmes focus on individual disciplines and are often aimed at those working in specific health care environments. The SPM programme transcends these boundaries taking recruits from nursing and the allied health professions and aims to prepare individuals to work in a range of settings in hospital and in the community, where people present with emergency or unscheduled care needs. However, the role mainly focuses on acute clinical assessment, physical examination, diagnosis and treatment of people who call 999 with a range of urgent and unscheduled care needs. In September 2009 there were over 720 SPMs in England, over 95 per cent of whom were paramedics registered with the HCPC (Bradley 2011) indicating that only 5 per cent are likely to come from a nursing background.

The focus of the SPM role is to enhance people's experience through their emergency care episode and to provide care that is service user-focused rather than system-focused. SPMs are trained to make autonomous decisions based on sound clinical assessment and judgement and to complete episodes of care in a range of settings when it is safe and appropriate to do so, and to arrange appropriate referrals when it is not. They will be sent to emergencies as a single responder and, depending on the nature of the emergency call, may be supported by an ambulance crew. SPMs form part of the flexible response to 999 calls. The majority of these calls are for a wide range of urgent and unscheduled medical, traumatic, health and social and mental health care conditions with only approximately 10 per cent of calls for life-threatening emergency conditions (Bradley 2005). Traditionally, around 70–77 per cent of calls result in admission to EDs; however, when SPMs are utilised, that number is reduced to 45–50 per cent (Mason, Knowles, Colwell *et al.* 2007, Woollard 2007). These figures support previous research identifying that up to 50 per cent of service users would be better managed in an alternative way to emergency department attendance (Bradley 2005). These statistics have been the main driver for development of this new role along with society's expectation that people with emergency and urgent needs receive more timely care in the most appropriate location for their clinical or social care need, with fewer handovers to other care professionals, and reduced use of the ambulance service, ED attendance and hospital admission.

CASE STUDY: Mary

Mary is a 76-year-old retired woman who lives with Rosie, her cat, in a house she has occupied since marrying her husband, Rob, 52 years ago. Rob died last year and Mary has been managing to live on her own with the support of her daughter 'popping in' occasionally.

Mary has a long-term medical problem, osteoarthritis of the knees and wrists, and is under the care of her general practitioner (GP). Mary is quite stoical about her condition and puts problems with pain, balance and occasional falls down to 'getting old'. These symptoms do affect her mobility and on bad days Mary just minimises her movements around the house. Mary doesn't like to worry her daughter too much because she thinks she has 'problems of her own' to worry about.

Recently Mary suffered a fall in her bathroom when she overbalanced picking up a towel from the floor. She sustained a wound to her forehead and was unable to get up from the floor or to get to the phone to seek assistance. She spent the night on the bathroom floor and was able to keep warm by pulling a pile of laundry from a low shelf onto herself.

In the morning an unanswered phone call from her daughter resulted in a 999 call to the ambulance service. John, a SPM in a rapid-response car, was dispatched to her assistance.

QUESTIONS

- What fears do you think Mary might have?
- How might John respond to those concerns?
- What options might be available to John in managing Mary's condition?

Falls are a significant cause of disability and a major health issue for older people (DH 2001) with over 400,000 attending the ED as a result and accounting for 10 per cent of calls (Halter, Close, Elrick *et al.* 2000).

In this case study, a traditional ambulance response to Mary's fall would usually result in transfer to the ED for wound assessment and closure; probably leading to admission for observation and an assessment of her ability to cope at home. Sending a SPM to Mary's assistance provides an increased range of treatment options and service user choice.

CASE STUDY continued

Upon arrival at the house, John introduces himself and commences an assessment of Mary's injuries and health status. The initial examination will focus on establishing whether or not she has any life-threatening or time-critical features and obtaining a focused history of what happened.

Having established that Mary has a head wound, John completes a full neurological assessment to help inform the diagnostic reasoning and clinical decision-making process.

Mary is worried about going into hospital. She is concerned about who will look after her cat, about being able to return to her own home and about an increase in dependence and disability.

QUESTIONS

- Does Mary really need to go into hospital?
- If Mary is admitted to hospital, what might the consequences be?
- What might John include in Mary's care plan if she is going to stay at home and who might be involved in this?

SPMs are able to provide a more enhanced assessment than a standard paramedic using the medical model for history taking and clinical examination and are also educated to undertake and consider an increased range of tests, treatment options and care pathways. Figure 16.1 illustrates the range of interprofessional referral options for the specialist paramedic. These include treatment for minor injuries and illness; care for exacerbations of chronic illness; and assessment of social care needs, falls and mental-health risk.

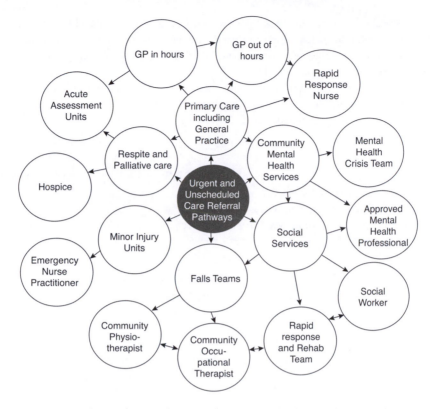

Figure 16.1 Range of interprofessional referral options for the specialist paramedic.

As referral to other health and social care professionals is such an important component of SPM practice, interpersonal skills, including assertiveness, negotiation and persuasion are key competencies for the SPM.

CASE STUDY continued

Following assessment, John cleanses Mary's head wound and uses a combination of wound glue and butterfly stitches to close the wound. John has established that Mary has no clinical need to attend the ED but now needs to be assured that she is safe to remain at home. With Mary's permission, John contacts her daughter who comes to discuss further care requirements. Having established that Mary overbalanced and fell but did not black out and collapse, John then commences a falls risk screening, checking for any cognitive impairment or any difficulties in balance or gait that might increase Mary's risk of falling again.

John concludes that Mary's occasional difficulties with balance mean she is at risk of further falls and, following discussion with Mary and her daughter, he makes a referral to the local Falls Prevention and Management Service; a joint initiative run by social services and the local Primary Care Trust as part of a Rapid Response and Rehabilitation Team. John discusses Mary's case with team member Jill, a community occupational therapist, who agrees to visit the following day. Mary's daughter says she will 'keep an eye on Mum' until then.

John advises them both how to keep the wound clean and when to remove the butterfly stitches. He then advises them what to do in case of any deterioration and documents a patient care record for forwarding to Mary's GP.

QUESTIONS

- How might Mary be feeling now?
- What concerns might Mary's daughter have?
- How important is it to involve Mary and her daughter in decisions about the best care?

ACTIVITY

Try to find out what community health and social care teams operate in your area.

The outcome for people who fall at home is better if they receive personalised care at home rather than transfer to hospital (Skelton 2006). Appropriate referral is important, as beyond the obvious and significant impact of injury, the effect of increased risk of further falls, loss of confidence, fear of falling, and restricted physical and social activity, have significant implications, not only to the individual, but also to society in general. Consequently it is important that appropriate engagement of primary and community care services occurs for service users who are not transported to hospital. A full assessment by a SPM should avoid the service user undergoing multiple assessments in different settings or by different health professionals (DH 2009).

CASE STUDY continued

The community occupational therapist and a colleague visited Mary at home the following day. They complete a multifactorial falls assessment involving a more intensive assessment than the screening process undertaken by John and identify specific, modifiable risk factors.

The assessment showed that Mary was at increased risk because of reduced mobility caused by her osteoarthritis and because of a number of hazards in her home. A care plan is established and over the ensuing weeks grab rails are installed at strategic points around the house, along with a toilet frame and shower stool. A community physiotherapist visits twice a week to do progressive balance and limb strengthening exercises to help improve Mary's mobility and to get her used to using a wheeled walking frame. Mary's daughter arranged for her to have a mobile alarm, a simple pendant worn around the neck which connects to a dedicated call centre that can be activated if she falls.

Six months after Mary's fall she continues to live independently with her cat, assisted by her daughter 'popping in' from time to time. Mary has not fallen again since. She said of her experience: 'that night I fell, I thought, this is it! I was really worried that I might have to go into a nursing home. Who would have looked after my cat? John was so kind and reassuring that day. Everyone who has helped me since has been the same. I can walk in my own garden and know that if I do fall again someone like John will come quickly to help me'.

QUESTIONS

- How might things have turned out differently if Mary had gone into hospital?
- How important were interpersonal skills in this case?

In this case, the SPM was able to complete a comprehensive assessment, resulting in treatment and referral on to another community provider avoiding unnecessary hospital attendance and admission. The government's National Director for Emergency Access has stated: 'The challenges for organisations in the provision of urgent care continue to be high profile and this care will no longer be provided just in emergency departments, or in General Practitioners surgeries' (SFH 2007: 9). While the SPM may be seen as an ideal solution for service users with urgent care needs, it has been recognised that services are still less than ideal. The National Audit Office (NAO 2011) identified that effectiveness relies on the availability of other services. Commissioners of such services are at different stages of developing electronic directories of services which can be used by practitioners to identify appropriate care pathways for service users. The SPM provides a rapid-response for service users in need of emergency or urgent care that is service user-focused, in the least intensive and most convenient and appropriate place for the service user: *their own home*. The development of this new role has been in response to a wider recognition that not all people accessing care via 999 calls require hospital attendance.

Perhaps it is best to view the SPM not only as a new role but also as an extension of an existing one. The key to the role's success is interprofessional working, as defined in Chapter 1. Our case study illustrates collaborative, interprofessional team work, with the SPM being both the first-contact healthcare provider and the gatekeeper to subsequent care.

Approved Mental Health Practitioner

In some instances changes to legislation herald changes that impact on roles and can remove the restrictions that limit duties and powers to particular professional groups. An example of this can be seen in the 2007 amendments to the England and Wales Mental Health Act 1983(2007) (MHA) (www.legislation.gov.uk). The amendments included important changes to the professionals eligible to perform various duties governed by this legislation, potentially having implications for interprofessional working and for service users and carers.

The main focus of this section of the chapter relates to the new role of the approved mental health practitioner (AMHP) which replaced the previous role of the Approved Social Worker (ASW). Changes relating to previous role of the Responsible Medical Officer, now called the Responsible Clinician, were also significant in terms of expanding roles. These roles are commonly seen in the context of a MHA assessment. This is where a service user presents with risks to their own or others' health and safety and a decision whether or not to detain them needs to be made. The assessment is typically undertaken by an AMHP, accompanied by the service user's Responsible Clinician and another doctor who is approved under the MHA or knows the patient well. It is not possible to discuss all the complexities of 1983 MHA and the amendments, but further details can be found in Brown (2010).

The role of the ASW under the original 1983 MHA, could only be undertaken by qualified registered social workers. This role was replaced by the AMHP giving rise to a new dawn whereby registered nurses, occupational therapists, chartered psychologists and existing ASWs could potentially undertake, what Bogg describes as arguably the most 'powerful civilian role in the UK' (2008: 115). The AMHP is responsible for deciding whether a MHA assessment is appropriate and coordinating all resources and aspects of that assessment. The AMHP will need to independently decide if someone should be detained in hospital against their will, even if this is recommended by the doctors. The Nearest Relative (a role included in s. 26 of the 1983(2007) MHA but not discussed in this chapter) also has the power to detain their relative, providing they have the two medical recommendations (see Hewitt 2009).

The creation of the AMHP role appeared to be an attempt to respond to various factors including the two mentioned below. First, concerns raised by the Association of Directors of Social Services relating to an ageing and retiring social work workforce and poor recruitment to the ASW role in some local authorities (Bailey 2012, Jones, Williams and Bayliss 2006). Second, the desire to utilise professionals within mental health teams differently by improving the skill mix and challenging powerful orthodoxies. A series of consultations with service users and carers reflected in the publications that advocated for new ways of working in mental health (DH 2007a, b, c) and the Mental Health Alliance (2007) put pressure on government for improved mental health services which reflected service user and carer need. Arising from this work the notion of Capable Teams was developed with widening roles (to include functions under the MHA) and increasing flexibility, effectiveness and competence.

Criteria, training and competencies

Although the eligibility to be an AMHP has been widened to other health professionals, the regulations (SO 2008) are clear that it remains the local authorities' responsibility to be satisfied that a person undertaking the role is competent in working with people with mental disorder. The local authority is the responsible body for commissioning regional AMHP training approved by the HCPC. This specialist training focuses on the values, knowledge and skills required to be competent and capable to undertake the role (GSCC 2010).

An eligible professional can apply to the local authority to undertake AMHP training. Prospective AMHPs need to have reached the appropriate level of professional competence in their own profession and have an understanding of the AMHP value base. If an applicant is successful they will be trained through a six-month postgraduate programme where they will need to demonstrate legal knowledge, academic competence and be assessed in practice (NIMHE 2007). Once warranted to practise an AMHP is required to complete 18 hours of approved local authority training a year. All AMHPs register with the HCPC and are required to adhere to the code of practice.

Writers such as Bogg (2008), Bailey (2012) and Laing (2012) express concerns that non-social work AMHPs may not come with social justice principles already established in their practice as the emphasis placed on these principles in preparatory education for social workers, as outlined by TCSW (2013), is not usually as strong for other professional groups. Hammick, Freeth, Copperman and Goodsman argue that there are 'similarities and differences in the professional values and ethical frameworks that practitioners in different professions work to' (2009: 26). However, the need for all mental health professionals to demonstrate a working knowledge of equalities and social justice issues has been expected since 2004 with the development of 'The Ten Essential Shared Capabilities for Mental Health Practice' (Hope 2004: 3) and endorsed by NIMHE (2007).

The AMHP needs to demonstrate knowledge of social perspectives of mental disorder as noted in the NIMHE (2007) guidance. It could be argued that maintaining a social perspective can be challenging to health professionals who may be more familiar with the 'medicalization' (Pollard 2010) of mental disorder. They may also have been professionally socialised into recognising the doctor as the lead clinician to whom they are subordinate. Golightley (2011) and Bailey (2012) argue that retaining the independence of the AMHP role is not only a legal necessity (under s. 13(2) of the MHA) but also vital if the AMHP is to offer a different perspective to the dominant medical perspective of mental disorder as the pathology of the individual. An eligible professional acquiring the skills to be an AMHP may first need to make what Miers (2010) describes as the internal adjustment necessary for acquiring new skills and values and may find what Oliver and Keeping (2010) suggest as their professional identity being in a state of flux. Therefore the need to explore these aspects is recognised in the AMHP training.

The AMHP needs training to ensure skills in interviewing, speaking with relatives and carers, gathering and scrutinising available information, balancing confidentiality and risk while working in collaboration with other agencies. This will enable the AMHP to make the most proportionate and least restrictive decision they can to mitigate the presenting risk and needs of the service users as explored by O'Gara (2008).

In the decision-making process it is imperative for the AMHP to understand the legal framework for their practice and the powers they are warranted to deploy. Knowledge of the Mental Health Act and the corresponding Code of

Practice (DH 2008) while essential, is not sufficient; the AMHP also needs to understand the duties conferred on them under the wider adult and child legislation by which they are bound (NIMHE 2007). Jones, Williams and Bayliss (2006) and Bailey (2012) reinforce these concerns highlighting the amount of legal knowledge that previous ASWs had to demonstrate in order to maintain their warrant. An informed understanding of how the Human Rights Act 1998 (www.legislation.gov.uk) influences decision making is also vital, so ensuring that this level of legal training is present in the AMHP training for non-social work AMHPs is essential. Writers such as Bogg (2008) see the additional Human Rights Act training gained as one among many positive outcomes of non-social work AMHPs undertaking this role, as potentially this understanding will filter into their everyday practice. Furthermore Jones *et al.* suggest that 'the AMHP being drawn from nursing and other professionals may add to the diversity and quality of the approved role' (2006).

Structural and organisational issues

At the time of writing, the AMHP role has existed for nearly 5 years. The majority of the existing ASW workforce converted to this new identity but despite the government's desire to see non-social work AMHPs in practice, estimates by the College of Social Work suggest that up until 2011 only around 121 were in practice nationally, compared with around 5,000 social work AMHPs (Bogg 2011). This may be due to a number of factors including structural and organisational issues, and the responsibilities of those who employ and approve AMHPs (NIMHE 2007). The local authority retained its responsibility to approve, warrant and ensure there are sufficient numbers of AMHPs and these functions cannot be delegated to any other organisation, including the NHS (NIMHE 2007). However, AMHPs do not necessarily have to be employed directly by the local authority, they can work for NHS, voluntary or private sector organisations. This raises the question as to why another organisation, such as the NHS, would wish to budget for their staff to train and undertake the work given that the provision of the AMHP service remains the local authority's responsibility. In practice this means that an individual AMHP could be in a complex contractual situation, with the local authority being responsible for their work as an AMHP even though they may be substantively employed elsewhere. This arrangement appears to require the AMHP to have a dual contract between the employing organisation and the local authority.

For social workers working within mental health services, becoming an ASW/AMHP was and is an expectation of their continuing professional development linked to pay and career development. Given the limited numbers of non-social work AMHPs this aspiration does not yet appear to be the case for other professional groups. This could be because they are not aware that they are eligible, combined with a lack of support or encouragement from their employer or, as suggested by Laing (2012), concerns in relation to the power and authority invested in the role. Also, in comparison to social workers, health professionals have negotiated more favourable pay and conditions. The lack of pay parity is likely to create tensions if remuneration for undertaking exactly the same role is not comparable (Jackson 2009, Jones *et al.* 2006). Therefore, the expectation that the AMHP role could widen the career pathways for non-social workers seems to still be progressing. The limited take-up from non-social workers illustrates that changes in legislation are not enough to change the workforce – more is needed in terms of awareness raising, support systems and incentives as well as reducing organisational boundaries.

CASE STUDY: Mrs Stanton

A community psychiatric nurse (CPN) in the local NHS Crisis Team has contacted the Adult Community Care Duty Desk to speak to an AMHP. The CPN wishes to make a referral for Mrs Stanton to be assessed under the MHA 2007.

Mrs Stanton's mental health is deteriorating and the CPN does not think it is safe for her to remain in the community as her mental illness is creating a risk to her own health and safety and that of others. As Mrs Stanton had told the CPN to leave the house, she is calling from her car.

Mrs Stanton is a single parent with a 13-year-old daughter who is at school but will be home within the hour. Mrs Stanton is also the primary carer for her mother who has dementia. Mrs Stanton had previously expressed concern as to who would look after their family dog if she needed to go into hospital.

QUESTIONS

- What knowledge do you think that the AMHP needs to intervene in this situation?
- What legislation is relevant to this situation?
- What difficulties do you think might arise as a result of the number of professionals who are involved in this situation?
- What differing perspectives do the interprofessional team bring to this situation?
- If you were subject to a MHA assessment what attributes, skills and competencies would you want the professionals involved in your assessment and care, to hold?
- Do you think any of these attributes, skills or competencies are restricted to a particular profession?

Conclusion

In their discussion of professional boundaries, Nancarrow and Borthwick (2005) make the point that the roles and boundaries of professionals have always changed and developed. Nancarrow and Borthwick provide a useful conceptual framework for considering types of changes identifying substitution (sometimes also called encroachment), diversification, horizontal and vertical substitution (2005). In the case of the AMHP role, one of the drivers for change was the shortage of social workers; so this can be seen as a horizontal substitution as those taking on the role are expected to be qualified and experienced practitioners who, irrespective of their professional background, undertake additional training to equip them for their new role. However, the SPM role can be seen as an example more of diversification as it is an extension of the paramedic role involving greater potential for treatment and care planning in situ. The SPM is able to prescribe and administer drugs that previously could only be administered by a medical professional so this could also be interpreted as vertical substitution. (The provision for suitably qualified and trained health professionals to prescribe certain medications is also considered in the medicine and physiotherapy chapters.)

Change and expansion of roles and boundaries are inevitable and happen all the time. Miers (2010) discusses development of professions and territories and how these adjust and change while Glasby and Dickinson (2008) consider how policy and organisational changes promoting partnership create changes that impact on individual roles and responsibilities and they question the extent to which change leads to better outcomes for users. One thing all professionals can be sure of is that change is inevitable; so as Hammick *et al.* (2009) and Thomas (Chapter 17) argue, practitioners need to be prepared for change and contribute to development.

RECOMMENDED READING

- Bailey D. (2012) *Interdisciplinary Working in Mental Health*. Basingstoke: Palgrave Macmillan.
- Bradley P. (2005) *Taking Healthcare to the Patient: Transforming NHS Ambulance Services*. London: DH.
- Bradley P. (2011) *Taking Healthcare to the Patient 2: A Review of 6 Years' Progress and Recommendations for the Future*. London: Association of Ambulance Chief Executives.
- Nancarrow S.A. and Borthwick A.M. (2005) Dynamic professional boundaries in the health care workforce. *Sociology of Health and Illness* **27**(7): 897–919.

References

Bailey D. (2012) *Interdisciplinary Working in Mental Health*. Basingstoke: Palgrave Macmillan.

Bogg D. (2008) *The Integration of Mental Health Social Work and the NHS, Post Qualifying Social Work Practice*. Exeter: Learning Matters.

Bogg D. (2011) National AMHP leads data. Unpublished survey, CSW.

Bradley P. (2005) *Taking Healthcare to the Patient: Transforming NHS Ambulance Services*. London: DH.

Bradley P. (2011) *Taking Healthcare to the Patient 2: A Review of 6 Years' Progress and Recommendations for the Future*. London: Association of Ambulance Chief Executives.

Brown R. (2010) *Post-Qualifying Social Work Practice: The Approved Mental Health Professionals Guide to Mental Health Law*. Exeter: Learning Matters.

DH (Department of Health) (2001) *National Service Framework for Older People*. London: DH.

DH (2007a) *New Ways of Working: A Best Practice Implementation Guide*. London: DH.

DH (2007b) *Mental Health: New Ways of Working for Everyone: Developing and Sustaining a Capable and Flexible Workforce*. London: DH.

DH (2007c) *Creating Capable Teams Approach (CCTA), Best Practice Guidance to Support the Implementation of New Ways of Working (NWW) and New Roles*. London: DH.

DH (2008) *Mental Health Act Code of Practice (2007)*. London: DH.

DH (2009) *Intermediate Care – Half Way Home: Updated Guidance for the NHS and Local Authorities*. London: DH.

Glasby J. and Dickinson H. (2008) *Partnership Working in Health and Social Care*. Bristol: Policy Press.

Golightley M. (2011) *Social Work and Mental Health Social Work Practice*. Exeter: Learning Matters.

GSCC (General Social Care Council) (2010) *Specialist Standard and Requirements for Post-Qualifying Social Work Education and Training*. London: GSCC.

Halter M., Close J.C., Elrick A., Brain G. and Swift C. (2000) *Falls in the Older Population: A Pilot Study to Assess those Individuals Who Are Attended to by the London Ambulance Service as a Result of a Fall but Are Not Conveyed to an Accident and Emergency Department*. London: Ambulance Service NHS Trust.

Hammick M., Freeth D., Copperman J. and Goodsman D. (2009) *Being Interprofessional*. Cambridge: Polity Press.

Hewitt D. (2009) *The Nearest Relative Handbook* (2nd edn). London: Jessica Kingsley.

Hope R. (2004) *The Ten Essential Shared Capabilities – A Framework for the Whole of the Mental Health Workforce*. London: NIMHE DH.

Jackson C. (2009) Approved mental health practitioner: Taking on the challenge of the role. *Mental Health Practice* **12**(8): 22–5.

Jones S., Williams B. and Bayliss M. (2006) Whose job is it anyway? *Mental Health Nursing*. www.blnz.com. Accessed April 2012.

Laing J. (2012) The Mental Health Act: exploring the role of nurses. *British Journal of Nursing* **21**(4): 234–8.

MA (Modernisation Agency) (2004) *Right Skill, Right Time, Right Place: The Emergency Care Practitioner Report*. London: DH.

Mason S., Knowles E., Colwell B., Dixon S., Wardrope J., Gorringe R., Snooks H., Perrin J. and Nicholls J. (*2007*) Effectiveness of paramedic practitioners in attending 999 calls from elderly people in the community: cluster randomised controlled trial. *British Medical Journal* **335**(7626): 919.

Mental Health Alliance (2007) Supporters campaign for a more rights-based Bill. **www**.mental-healthalliance.org.uk. Accessed May 2012.

Miers M. (2010) Learning for new ways of working. In Pollard K.C., Thomas J. and Miers M. (eds), *Understanding Interprofessional Working in Health and Social Care: Theory and Practice*. Basingstoke: Palgrave Macmillan, pp. 74–89.

Nancarrow S.A. and Borthwick A.M. (2005) Dynamic professional boundaries in the health care workforce. *Sociology of Health and Illness* **27**(7): 897–919.

NAO (National Audit Office) (2011) *Transforming NHS Ambulance Services*. London: SO.

NIMHE (National Institute for Mental Health in England) (2007) *Mental Health Act 2007 New Roles*. London: NIMHE.

O'Gara J. (2008) Best practice in emergency mental health social work: on using good judgement. In Jones K., Cooper B. and Ferguson H. (eds), *Best Practice in Social Work: Critical Perspectives*. Basingstoke: Palgrave Macmillan, pp. 213–234.

Oliver B. and Keeping C. (2010) Individual and professional identity. In Pollard K.C., Thomas J. and Miers M. (eds), *Understanding Interprofessional Working in Health and Social Care: Theory and Practice*. Basingstoke: Palgrave Macmillan, pp. 90–104.

Pollard K.C. (2010) Medicalization thesis. In Pollard K.C., Thomas J. and Miers M. (eds) *Understanding Interprofessional Working in Health and Social Care: Theory and Practice*. Basingstoke: Palgrave Macmillan, pp. 121–37.

SFH (Skills for Health) (2007) *The Competence and Curriculum Framework for the Emergency Care Practitioner*. Bristol: SFH.

Skelton D. (2006) Preventing falls in older people. *Practice Nurse* **32**(1): 22–4.

SO (Stationery Office) (2008) *The Mental Health (Approved Mental Health Professionals) (Approval) (England) Regulations*, London: SO.

TCSW (2013) *Professional Capabilities Framework.* www.tcsw.org.uk. Accessed October 2013.

WAS (Welsh Ambulance Service) (2011) *Getting There: Annual Report 2009–10.* St Asaph: WAS NHS Trust.

Woollard M. (2007) Specialist paramedics and emergency admissions. *British Medical Journal* **335**(7626): 893–4.

17

Issues for the Future

Judith Thomas

Introduction

This chapter draws together some of the themes and issues relating to inter-professional working (IPW) that emerge from this book. The areas considered cover personal issues relating to the impact on individual workers, the local context within which they work and broader issues of policy. The following themes are identified for further consideration.

- *Continued change and uncertainty.* Policies and practices in health, social care, education, criminal justice and housing are constantly changing and developing. Since the first edition of this book and while writing this edition changes have been announced to the structure of some services and the way they are organised. The pace of change means that practitioners now, more than ever, need to have the capacity for critical reflection and the ability to constantly update and review their knowledge and skills.
- *So what's new about IPW?* This theme explores what is new and different about this topic in the 21st century and the implications for workers and service delivery.
- *Service user and carers.* Here the importance of service users and carers being at the centre of service development, care planning and evaluation, rather than being passive recipients, is identified. However, the challenges of making this a reality are considerable requiring a fundamental rethink of many taken-for-granted practices and assumptions.
- *Roles.* New roles are emerging prompting questions relating to professional identity, management, support and supervision and existing roles are becoming increasingly complex and blurred.

■ *Interprofessional and professional identity.* Inherent in initiatives from recent policies are potential mixed messages that need highlighting, one example being, the strengthening of professional identity through protection of titles and registration whilst simultaneously promoting IPW.

■ *Professional education and development.* The chapter concludes by offering a format for practitioners to use that promotes critical reflection of IPW.

Exploring the tensions, contradictions and paradoxes within these themes helps identify why IPW is necessary and desirable but also why it can be problematic. In this chapter it is argued that IPW needs to be a conscious and explicit process leading to collaborative working between service users, carers and professionals. Questions for practitioners are posed to promote reflective analysis, greater understanding and critical evaluation of their own attitudes to collaboration and the way in which IPW operates.

Continued change and uncertainty

In Chapters 4–16 authors identify how each profession has developed, they discuss recent trends and consider the continuing evolution of their discipline illustrating how IPW is constructed in many different ways. It can be formal or informal, it ranges from different professionals working in separate teams coming together in order to respond to the needs of individual service users to integrated teams that consist of many different professionals. The extent of IPW in different situations can be seen as being on a continuum. In straightforward situations, IPW may involve some initial joint planning and shared record keeping. Where people have more complex needs, workers, service users and carers will need to engage in a more active and conscious way. Each situation is likely to need a different level of IPW and this will vary over time. Professionals need to recognise the level of interdependence required to deliver services effectively and be flexible about how this can best be achieved.

The changes in policy and legislation articulated throughout the book illustrate how IPW is continuing to evolve and the impact this has on how services are organised. The chapters on youth work, physiotherapy and social work refer to social enterprises that have now taken on the delivery of some services, general practitioners can now provide and commission services and private companies are increasingly providing services from domiciliary care to criminal justice. Perhaps the only thing professionals can be certain of is that services and practices will continue to change and develop.

QUESTIONS

■ Choose one of the health and social care professions from Part II of this book. Using the relevant chapter and the references provided identify any significant changes since the year 2000 noted by the authors.

■ What impact might these changes have on service users, carers and the workers involved?

■ What additional changes can you identify that have occurred since this book was published?

So what's new about interprofessional working?

As asserted in Chapter 1, IPW is not new. Some contact between different professionals in their daily work has always occurred but practices that have existed formally and informally for decades as each profession has emerged are being actively constructed, named and defined. Despite attempts for closer definitions, different terms describing collaborative practice are often used interchangeably. Whittington, Thomas and Quinney (2009) discuss the different terminology and use the term 'Interprofessional and Inter-agency Collaboration' (IPIAC) to convey the need for different levels of collaboration between agencies and professionals.

Marsh and Fisher (1992) identify the dangers of the DATA (*do all that already*) where workers assume they are adopting particular practices. IPW may have existed for some time but current policy and financial drivers together with well-publicised failures mean it needs to be an explicit and conscious activity integrated in the practice of all health and social care professionals. While there have been developments in policy, procedures and legislation, for example in relation to children as outlined in Chapter 11, these structures are not enough and working collaboratively needs to be a core capability of everyone. Darzi (DH 2008) highlights the importance of individual responsibility not only for one's own work but also for that of the team.

================================ **ACTIVITY** ================================

Think of a situation where you have assumed you *do all that already* in relation to IPW. What systems could you use more actively or develop with colleagues to support effective IPW? This might include, for example, reviewing the collaboration within each piece of work you undertake, using team meetings to discuss collaborative working practices or setting up a peer review process with a colleague from another discipline.

Chapter 2 considers the difficulties for individual workers and some of the conflicts, stresses and opportunities that IPW may present. There are myriad factors that influence how individual workers feel about IPW. The way in which changes have been implemented at local level will affect the enthusiasm or otherwise of the workforce. In interprofessional teams the leader may be drawn from one of a number of disciplines. This can create additional tension for workers who may feel isolated and consider their unique professional skills are not being developed through supervision. They may also feel that their particular professional perspectives are being diffused or eroded. In many situations staff will have made deliberate choices to move from uniprofessional to IPW and embrace the accompanying challenges. Others will have started their careers in integrated teams so likely to have been socialised into IPW.

Professionals emerging from training will have experienced varying emphasis on IPW in their programmes. In some programmes students will have opportunities to learn with and from other professionals, as can been seen from the examples provided on the CAIPE website (www.caipe.org.uk). Reviews of research (for example Barr, Koppel, Reeves *et al.* 2005, Hammick, Freeth Koppel *et al.* 2007, Reeves, Zwarenstein, Goldman *et al.* 2010) show that the link between interprofessional learning and improved interprofessional collaboration in practice is difficult to evaluate and more systematic research is needed. However, practitioners in studies by Derbyshire and Machin (2011) and Pollard, Miers and Rickaby (2012) and studies cited in Barr, Helme and D'Avray (2011) indicate that interprofessional learning had helped to prepare them to work effectively with colleagues from other disciplines.

ACTIVITY

Develop your knowledge of other professions.

- Identify the professions you are likely to work with in a specified setting, for example a nursing home, a summer play scheme, a community team working with people with learning disabilities.
- Assess your knowledge of the professional roles and boundaries of each one on a basis of a scale of 1–3, where 1 represents very limited knowledge, 2 represents some awareness but gaps in knowledge, and 3 represents very well informed.

Name of Profession   Your score
     (1–3)

a)

b)

c)

If the professions you have identified are included in Part II of this book, read the relevant chapter(s). You could also ask a representative from those professions to talk to you about their roles, responsibilities and professional boundaries and use the opportunity to share information about your own profession.

Assess your attitudes to interprofessional working.

Which of the statements below most closely reflects your attitude to IPW:

1 ambivalent
2 willing
3 see as essential.

If you have identified yourself as category 1 you will find it useful to read the section on willing participation in Chapter 2 and also look at the 'Shaping our lives' website (www.shapingourlives.org.uk) which offers service user perspectives on the value of integrated care. Whatever way you have responded it is also worth thinking about what makes IPW problematic, as this will help you to deepen your understanding of some of the challenges. It may also help you think about ways of developing your own practice and that of your team. In the Cameron, Lart, Bostock and Coomber (2012) literature review of IPW they identify financial uncertainty, constant reorganisation, different professional philosophies and lack of trust and respect as factors that hinder joint working. While you may not be able to do much about some of the contextual or organisational factors, being aware of these and discussing them with colleagues may be helpful in avoiding blame and potentially can lead to some collective action to influence the direction of change. Exploring the impact on service users of aspects such as lack of trust and articulating similarities and differences between professionals to develop common aims will help to promote collaborative working. The studies in Cameron et al. (2012) identified the importance of having regular team-building opportunities and using supervision or team meetings to enhance communication, information sharing and joint working.

Policy developments that promote IPW are identified in Chapter 1 but the extent to which these initiatives have filtered down to frontline working has for some time been recognised as being variable. Irvine, Kerridge, McPhee and Freeman, citing reviews of the empirical literature, argue that 'relationships between service providers remain variable and complicated' (2002: 199). The impact of this for workers and service users is highlighted in Chapter 8, illustrating the sorts of gaps in services that can occur when national policy advocates changes from specialised services to more integrated approaches.

Policy changes take time to permeate everyday practice particularly when the pace and scale of change is as radical as in the late 1990s and the early years of the 21st century. Charlesworth draws attention to the problems associated with the 'possibility of "too much" partnership and consultation which can also slow down organisations' progress on meeting local targets' (2001: 283). She highlights the paradox that can occur:

> the government wants partnership to happen but this, added to the scale and pace of change, targets and performance measures, means there is an element of retreat to core business and it is still too early for organisations to see partnership working itself as core business. Thus there are a number of conflicting tensions and pressures which are potentially proving counterproductive to government policy on joined-up working.
>
> (Charlesworth 2001: 285)

It is still difficult to assess the impact of policies that advocate for IPW, as noted by Cameron *et al.* (2012) who draw attention to the difficulty of finding studies that clearly identify the impact of policy changes.

IPW requires new thinking about leadership. The case for non-hierarchical structures has been argued extensively (see Chapter 2). However, the NHS and local authorities, where the majority of health and social care workers have traditionally been employed, are bureaucracies with hierarchical structures. This prompts questions as to whether the argument for fewer hierarchies in IPW is naive and unworkable and whether it is unrealistic to deny real differences between professional practices. Structural differences in status created by pay differentials, entry requirements for training, level of qualification, political power of professional associations and historical standing cannot be denied and all contribute to the maintenance of traditional power relationships. At local level, agency policies and team practices may create more equitable ways of working where power differences are minimised and the valuable contribution of all team members, including service users and carers, is recognised. Chapter 2 discusses the complexities of power and provides a useful format for analysing it. An appreciation of power and how this connects with structural inequalities, together with the opportunities to openly consider how this potentially and actually permeates relationships, may help practitioners and teams toward greater collaboration.

Service users and carers

Improving services for users and carers has for some time, as reflected in the NHS and Community Care Act 1990 (www.legislation.gov.uk) been part of the rationale for IPW and Chapter 3 explores the more recent realities and limitations of this. Obviously there are challenges for all professionals in making partnership a reality and ensuring that service users have some control, as illustrated by the case studies in this book. In Chapter 6, the doctor has to determine the degree of risk if Mr Fitzpatrick stays at home and face a potential public outcry if problems then occur. Chapter 12 identifies motivation as a key factor in the work of probation officers, but service users are offenders so their use of the service may be compulsory with limited choice between using the service or being in prison. Here the notion of the service user being in control is inevitably constrained. One of the criticisms in the Laming Report (2003) (see Chapter 11) was that none of the professionals spoke directly to Victoria Climbié about her life or how she was feeling, so even the basics of user involvement were absent. In Chapter 4, Sofie's mother, as the carer, experienced difficulty challenging professional viewpoints. The obstacles she faced in finding out about options relating to medical procedures and the fight she had to promote the value of sign language so that her daughter was included in communications are typical of the sorts of frustrations that carers can experience.

================================ **QUESTIONS** ================================

■ Identify a situation where you have been a service user or a carer.
■ To what extent did you feel in control?
■ In what ways was the power or control you had in the situation limited?
■ How could your involvement have been enhanced?

The way in which health and social care services were set up in 1948 with separate funding streams that translated into different eligibility criteria led to frequent conflict as to who was responsible for the funding of services and, as discussed by Vatcher and Jones in Chapter 14, these tensions still exist. Service users and carers suffered most from this situation being passed 'from one service to another in the hope that the cost will be met from an alternative source' (Barton 2003: 113). Changes have been made in the way funding is allocated, as discussed in Chapters 1 and 14, for example direct payments have been introduced giving service users access to funding to buy in their own care. Consequently the way in which money can now be allocated is an important step in giving service users and carers more power and control over their lives; however, professionals have a responsibility to work together and with service users and carers to support this process.

Roles

In Chapter 2, the importance of clarity and competence in one's own professional role for effective IPW is discussed. Other chapters illustrate different views within professions and externally about their role and purpose. For example, within social work there has long been a debate about whether they are agents of state control whose purpose is to help people fit into existing structures or whether through community and political action they should be attempting to change society (Barnes and Hugman 2002). In Chapter 11, Kennison and Fletcher highlight differences between public perceptions of what the police should be doing and the view of the police endorsing targets set by government that, in turn, determine levels of funding. In Chapter 7, the complexity of the midwife's role and the blend of knowledge and skills needed for competent practice is considered. This may include, for example, detailed physiological knowledge of pregnancy and birthing combined with an understanding of the potential psychological reactions, social conditions and the skills to promote the rights of the woman whilst ensuring the health of the baby. From these discussions we see that the role of each professional is complex and requires a blend of different types of knowledge and skills; roles are not fixed but depend on the context within which the person is working. Understanding of the role of others is an important aspect of IPW; however, it is also crucial to appreciate, as discussed in the previous chapter, that boundaries around roles are changing and some role overlap in interprofessional teams is inevitable. The ability to clarify and negotiate roles and to be able to articulate these clearly to service users and carers is an essential capability of any professional.

QUESTIONS

Choose a professional group and identify some of the potential tensions for the workers in that profession, others they may work with, service users and carers in terms of the way in which their role could be perceived.

- What stereotypes do you have of each profession?
- How were these formed?
- How are they perpetuated?
- What purpose do they serve?

Changes to the role of each professional and the activities they perform are a common feature of modern health and social care services, as discussed in Chapter 16. One example is of prescribing medication; until recently this responsibility rested with doctors but now in some instances, suitably trained nurses prescribe from a specified list of medications, with this function being extended to physiotherapists and others as discussed in Chapters 6 and 10.

Interprofessional and professional identity

Alongside moves towards role flexibility and new ways of working there is also greater emphasis on professional identity. Indications of this include the legal protection of titles of registered nurse, social worker or physiotherapist. While there has been long-standing protection in some cases, such as doctor, others are more recent with provision made for protection of the title of social worker and physiotherapist introduced in 2004. National Occupational Standards, Codes of Ethics and academic benchmarks for qualifications have been developed in profession-specific ways. Whilst these documents include reference to collaboration and understanding the contribution of others, they have mainly evolved from within the discipline to which they refer. It could also be argued that they make the distinction between different professions more acute and that this potentially militates against IPW. However, there is broader debate in the literature about this, with some authors maintaining that a strong professional identity serves as a solid foundation for IPW (see, for example, Kenny 2002).

Additionally, as discussed in the previous chapter, we are now seeing specific roles with legal status that transcend a specific professional identity, such as the approved mental health practitioner, the responsible clinician and the specialist paramedic, that have replaced and extended previous roles to allow a wider range of professionals to carry out the associated responsibilities. While paths have been paved for certain roles to move beyond a specific professional identity, the motivation to take on these roles has been limited, perhaps illustrating Cameron's (2011) assertion that some of the human and social aspects of these changes have not been fully considered.

Organisations such as NICE (the National Institute for Health and Clinical Excellence) and SCIE (the Social Care Institute for Excellence) that support professionals in developing and disseminating research to inform practice have been established. These organisations were funded by government to provide information and guidance for practitioners, service users, patient and carers on different treatments and working practices. They also provide useful resources to support IPW, for example, those by Cameron *et al.* (2012) and Whittington *et al.* (2009). Professional bodies support and monitor standards within each profession, for example the NMC for nursing and midwifery, GMC for medicine and the HCPC for professions such as physiotherapy, occupational therapy and social work. These initiatives, together with points about the status of different professions, as argued in Chapter 2, all contribute to a clearer professional identity.

Arguments presented in Chapter 1 and made by others (for example, Ahmad and Broussine 2003, Harle Page and Ahmad 2010) also warn that increasing levels of centralised government and managerial control, together with the effect of performance targets, undermine professional choice. While the blurring of boundaries in some areas may be positive (for example, assessment no longer being the preserve of social work or probation) it also creates concerns about the demise of professional identity and undermines liberal values.

Professional education and development

Whittington considers

> The ethical responsibility of …care professionals is not only 'to do' as effectively as their skills with allow, but also to 'reflect' as rigorously as possible both on what they do and what is being offered as evidence to justify it.

> (2003: 30)

Such views can be traced back to Schön who argues that professionals are consistently faced with problems where one theory or solution cannot easily be applied and suggests skilled professional workers actually draw on a range of theories to help them make sense of their world. He also questions whether 'the prevailing concepts of professional education will ever yield a curriculum adequate to the complex, unstable, uncertain, and conflictual worlds of practice' (1987: 12). So while professional training may help people understand and analyse their role and ensure they have relevant knowledge for practice, it is unrealistic to assume professionals will qualify with all the knowledge they need for each situation they will encounter. This combined with the instability created by the changing nature of policy, partly prompted by political changes, and factors such as variations in demography and social structures means, as Hammick, Freeth, Copperman and Goodsman (2009) highlight, that professionals need to be equipped and motivated to critically reflect regularly on their working practices.

The questions provided below can be used to consider, explore, analyse and evaluate IPW. They can be used by teams to explore collective practices or by individuals to critically reflect on their own work. However, as IPW takes place in a social context and requires interaction with others, discussion with other team members is encouraged. In working through the questions you will need to focus on a particular incident or situation; this way of reflecting on an incident using a structured format is often referred to as a Critical Incident Analysis (see Taylor 2000 and Thomas 2004). The questions provided are designed to prompt thinking and reflection, consequently some will not have clear, easy answers or solutions.

ACTIVITY

Critical Incident Analysis:

Start by thinking generally about the context in which you are working and the strengths and limitations of IPW in this setting.

Think of an example of some work either with a specific service user or carer or an event, such as a meeting, where you observed or were part of IPW.

- What were your first impressions of IPW in relation to the incident?

- What was effective about the way different professions worked together?

- What hindered IPW?

- Where did this happen? (details of room, setting, physical environment and so on).

- What did you notice about the way people *communicated* with each other?
    - Did everyone who wanted to, contribute to the discussion?
    - Was anyone excluded or ignored?
    - Did anyone dominate? If so, how and why?
    - What did you notice about the non-verbal communication?
    - What did you notice about the use of language – was it specialised?
- Was there any profession or person missing who could have made a useful contribution?

- What did you notice about the relationships between those involved? Was there any particularly strong connection or rapport between particular people?

- What were the service user's and carer's views, expertise and strengths?
  - How central were they to the discussion?

- What was the atmosphere like? (such as conflict, humour, routines, refreshments and so on).

- What was the main content of the discussion?

  - Diagnosis/identification of problems, progress, future planning?
  - Did any of the discussion consider how professions had or could potentially work together?

- What was your role?
  - How clear were you about this?
  - What role conflicts did you experience or observe?
  - Did you understand the role of others present?
  - If not, why not and what can you do about this?

- Which of the following skills did you use and how effectively did you use them?
  - Active listening
  - Sharing your views
  - Being aware of other people
  - Using eye contact
  - Using silences
  - Summarising
  - Asking open questions
  - Acknowledging other contributions
  - Challenging.

- How did power and leadership operate?
  - Was there a formal leader and if so why did this person take the lead?
  - Were there any shifts or changes in leadership during the process, if so why?
  - What were the power dynamics? (use Table 2.1 in Chapter 2 to help you analyse these).
  - What did you notice about the way in which formal and informal power operated?
  - How did you use your power and influence?
  - Did you feel able to challenge others?
  - Were any viewpoints or contributions ignored or undermined?
  - Was there conflict, if so how was this resolved?
  - What else did you notice about power?

- What learning occurred?
  - For you?
  - For others?
  - How did this happen? (for example, discussion in group, follow-up discussion with practice teacher, mentor, supervisor, clinical educator and so on).

- Did any new practices or ways of working emerge from the situation?

- How can you apply the understanding you have gained from this situation in the future?

- What gaps in your knowledge, understanding and skills can you identify and how can you bridge these?

Follow your learning through into action by identifying who you may need to talk to, what you might need to investigate further and what skills you might need to practise. Also consider how you will take forward your insights into interprofessional practice arising from this incident, for example, you may want to write a letter to a senior manager, discuss key points in a team meeting or arrange to meet again with the other people involved in the incident to share perspectives.

Conclusion

The challenges of IPW need to be recognised. Reason considered that working in multidisciplinary teams is

> very difficult ... it requires highly evolved practitioners who are in significant ways non-attached to their paradigms of practice and to their Self. More than this it requires a social setting which supports and encourages such detachment: an evolved multidisciplinary group.
>
> (1996: 245)

These challenges are still apparent today and consequently IPW will not happen unless people are committed to identifying and working through difficulties as they occur. Policy initiatives and the needs of those who use services and resources will continue to steer the interprofessional agenda. In order for new policies to operate effectively they need the commitment of professionals to work collaboratively with the ability to critically evaluate practices and develop these with service users and carers. The chapter authors in this book have conveyed the complexity of incorporating collaboration within the context of distinct professional roles. The task has stimulated authors to think more deeply about their personal paradigms of practice and the integration of interprofessional identity within their specific uniprofessional culture. It is hoped this book will help readers to think critically about the nature of interprofessional practice and how this can be incorporated into their daily work.

RECOMMENDED READING

■ Hammick M., Freeth D., Copperman J. and Goodsman D. (2009) *Being Interprofessional*. Cambridge: Polity Press.

■ *Journal of Interprofessional Care* – this publication covers aspects of interprofessional working for a range of disciplines drawing on national and international research studies. http://informahealthcare.com. Accessed February 2013.

■ Littlechild B. and Smith R. (eds) (2012) *A Handbook for Interprofessional Practice in the Human Services: Learning to Work Together*. Harlow: Pearson.

References

Ahmad Y. and Broussine M. (2003) The UK public sector modernization agenda: reconciliation and renewal? *Public Management Review* 5(1): 45–62.

Barnes D. and Hugman R. (2002) Portrait of social work. *Journal of Interprofessional Care* **16**: 277–88.

Barr H., Helme M. and D'Avray L. (2011) *Developing Interprofessional Education in Health and Social Care Courses in the United Kingdom.* Paper 12. The Higher Education Academy, Health Sciences and Practice. www.health.heacademy.ac.uk. Accessed June 2013.

Barr H., Koppel I., Reeves S., Hammick M. and Freeth D. (2005) *Effective Interprofessional Education: Argument, Assumption and Evidence.* Oxford: Blackwell.

Barton C. (2003) Allies and enemies: the service user as care co-ordinator. In Weinstein J., Whittington C. and Leiba T. (eds) *Collaboration in Social Work Practice.* London: Jessica Kingsley Publications, pp. 103–20.

Cameron A. (2011) Impermeable boundaries? Developments in professional and inter-professional practice. *Journal of Interprofessional Care* **25**: 53–8.

Cameron A., Lart R., Bostock L. and Coomber C. (2012) *Research Briefing 41: Factors that Promote and Hinder Joint and Integrated Working between Health and Social Care Services.* London: SCIE.

Charlesworth J. (2001) Negotiating and managing partnership in primary care. *Health and Social Care in the Community* **9**(5): 279–85.

Derbyshire J.A. and Machin A.I. (2011) Learning to work collaboratively: nurses' views of their pre-registration interprofessional education: implications for theory and practice. *Nurse Education in Practice* **11**(4): 239–44.

DH (Department of Health) (2008) *High Quality Care for All: NHS Next Stage Review Final Report.* Chair Lord Darzi. London: The Stationery Office.

Hammick M., Freeth D., Copperman J. and Goodsman D. (2009) *Being Interprofessional* Cambridge: Polity Press.

Hammick M., Freeth D., Koppel I., Reeves S. and Barr H. (2007) A best evidence systematic review of interprofessional education: BEME Guide no 9. *Medical Teacher* **29**(8): 735–51.

Harle T., Page M. and Ahmad Y. (2010) Organisational Issues. In Pollard K.C., Thomas J. and Miers M. (eds) *Understanding Interprofessional Working in Health and Social Care: Theory and Practice.* Basingstoke: Palgrave Macmillan, pp. 138–55.

Irvine R., Kerridge I., McPhee J. and Freeman S. (2002) Interprofessionalism and ethics: consensus or clash of cultures? *Journal of Interprofessional Care* **16**: 199–210.

Laming, Lord (2003) *Inquiry into the Death of Victoria Climbié.* London: The Stationery Office.

Kenny G. (2002) Children's nursing and interprofessional collaboration: challenges and opportunities. *Journal of Clinical Nursing* **11**(3): 306–13.

Marsh P. and Fisher M. (1992) *Good Intentions: Developing Partnership in Social Services.* York: Joseph Rowntree Foundation.

Pollard K.C., Miers M. and Rickaby C. (2012) 'Oh why didn't I take more notice?' Professionals' views and perceptions of pre-qualifying preparation for interprofessional working in practice. *Journal of Interprofessional Care* **26**(5): 355–61.

Reason P. (1996) Power and conflict in multidisciplinary collaboration. In Patrick C. and Pietroni C. (eds) *Innovation in Community Care and Primary Health.* New York: Churchill Livingston, pp. 237–46.

Reeves S., Zwarenstein M., Goldman J., Barr H., Freeth D., Koppel I. and Hammick M. (2010) The effectiveness of interprofessional education: key findings from a new systematic review. *Journal of Interprofessional Care* **24**(3): 230–41.

Schön D.A. (1987) *Educating the Reflective Practitioner.* San Francisco: Jossey-Bass.

Taylor B.J. (2000) *Reflective Practice: A Guide for Nurses and Midwives.* Buckingham: Open University Press.

Thomas J. (2004) Using 'Critical Incident Analysis' to promote critical reflection and holistic assessment. In Gould N. and Baldwin M. (eds), *Social Work, Critical Reflection and the Learning Organisation.* Aldershot: Ashgate, pp. 101–16.

Whittington C. (2003) Collaboration and partnership in context. In Weinstein J., Whittington C. and Leiba T. (eds), *Collaboration in Social Work Practice*. London: Jessica Kingsley, pp. 13–18.

Whittington C., Thomas J. and Quinney A. (2009) *Interprofessional and Inter Agency Collaboration*. eLearning resource Social Care Institute for Excellence. www.scie.org.uk/. Accessed November 2012.

Index